THE NON-VERBAL CHILD

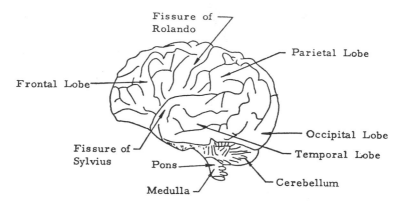

VIEW OF LEFT SIDE OF ADULT HUMAN BRAIN

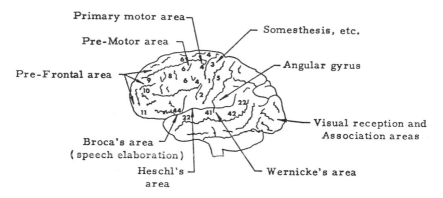

BRODMANN'S NUMBERINGS OF CEREBRAL CORTEX

(Second Printing)

THE
NON-VERBAL CHILD

By

SOL ADLER, Ph.D.

*Professor of Health Education, and
Director of the Speech and Hearing Clinic
East Tennessee State University
Johnson City, Tennessee*

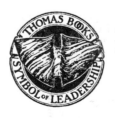

CHARLES C THOMAS • PUBLISHER

Springfield · Illinois · U.S.A.

Published and Distributed Throughout the World by

CHARLES C THOMAS • PUBLISHER

BANNERSTONE HOUSE

301-327 East Lawrence Avenue, Springfield, Illinois, U.S.A.

NATCHEZ PLANTATION HOUSE

735 North Atlantic Boulevard, Fort Lauderdale, Florida, U.S.A.

First Printing, 1964
Second Printing, 1966

*With THOMAS BOOKS careful attention is given to all details of
manufacturing and design. It is the Publisher's desire to present books
that are satisfying as to their physical qualities and artistic possibilities
and appropriate for their particular use. THOMAS BOOKS will be true
to those laws of quality that assure a good name and good will.*

Printed in the United States of America
W-2

DEDICATION

To my wife, Betty, and our children:
Gay Suzette, Gerald Scott, Pauline
Alisa, Deborah Lynn, and
Karen Elizabeth

PREFACE

THERE IS NEED for a textbook that will present a clinical approach to the problems of the non-verbal child who may also manifest other handicapping conditions. Such a book should help the student to understand:

(a) The psycho-dynamics involved in the sequential organization of communicative behavior.

(b) The possible causes of dysfunctions and their differential diagnosis.

(c) A multi-disciplined approach to habilitation.

This book is an outgrowth of such a need. It is designed for the relatively unsophisticated student or habilitationist who is concerned with the many problems his patient might have, but who has not had the training to determine exactly what these needs are and what to do about them.

It is better, of course, if an interdisciplinary team can tackle such problems, but unfortunately, such a team is rarely available. "Referrals" are another and more common way of coping with the problems of the multi-handicapped child. However, the therapist must first be aware of the need for such a referral, and must have a referral source available, as well as parental cooperation. Quite commonly one or more of these factors are inoperative. All too often a therapist must "be everything" and "do everything" if his patient is to be helped.

We envision the day when training centers will train "communication" therapists who are well versed in all of the habilitative specialities. As of now, however, because of the fragmented programs that so often exist, there is little formalized training in all of the different skills needed to habilitate the non-verbal child. There are, moreover, few or no textbooks that integrate the clinical skills necessary for such a habilitative program and this book is meant to serve this purpose.

We have tried to keep this book free from theoretical entanglements; our whole aim has been to make this a practical *guide* for the habilitationist. We would like to emphasize that this book is only intended to survey the various problems.

We have deliberately omitted much detail when we thought it was too theoretical or too argumentative. Also omitted are therapeutic specialities that, in our opinion, are too specialized for inclusion in such a text. Certainly such omissions of content and discipline are disputable, but in our opinion their inclusion would have defeated our goal—a simple yet over-all clinical picture of the non-verbal child.

ACKNOWLEDGMENT

Acknowledgment and thanks are extended to all my students, past and present, for their questions, criticisms, and papers; to my secretary, Janice Bennett, for service "above and beyond"; to my colleagues, and, in particular to Professors Richard Cornell, Mary V. Dickerson, and Walter Mitchell for a stimulating environment and helpful advice.

S. A.

CONTENTS

THE NON-VERBAL CHILD

Chapter I

INTRODUCTION

T HERE IS A sequence of events involved in the development of one's communicative abilities. These events are not autonomous but are dependent upon each other as they develop. Any impairment in this overlapping-interacting chain of events may affect not only a specific function, but also, in varying degrees, the other functions inherent in communicative development.

These events include the following: (1) end organ sensation —the ability to sense the experiences offered by one's environment and to make the proper adjustments to these experiences; (2) perceptual learning—the ability to recognize and discriminate these sensations and to learn from one's responses to them; (3) conceptual development—the ability to abstract similarities from among different perceptions and categorize or classify them; (4) symbolic development—allows for the communication of ideas, emotions, and desires through a language consisting of signs, signals, or words. (All of these preceding functions allow for cognitive development—the meaningful use of information in problem-solving situations.) (5) neuro-motor development— allows for the selection of appropriate motor patterns and for the refinement of muscle tonus; (6) muscular responses—allows for the appropriate response; (7) feedback system—allows the response to be scanned and analyzed by our brain, and corrected if necessary. These responses are modified by our affective (mood), conative (will), and psychomotor behavior as well as our judgments, insights, and personality.

It is important that the habilitationist remember that depressed functioning of any one part of the chain may affect, to varying degrees, all other parts of the chain. Although our focal point in this book is the language development of the non-verbal child, this child may also manifest other problems of concern to the habilitationist.

There are four basic causes of non-verbalism, each of which may also affect other parts of the sequential chain. These causes are: brain-injury, mental subnormality, emotional illness, and deafness.

It is important that the habilitationist be able to correctly diagnose the cause of the disordered functioning in addition to

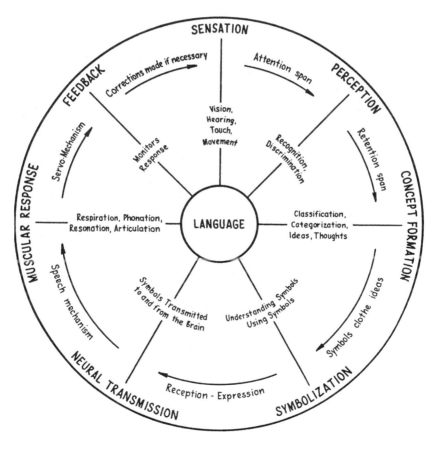

LANGUAGE WHEEL

recognizing the types of disordered functioning that are present. To do this, the examiner must be familiar with the various symptomatologies and have appropriate tests at his disposal. Above all, however, the examiner must have an over-all picture of the problem and recognize the need that so often exists for an all-inclusive therapy program incorporating all of the various therapies that might be of benefit to the child.

Chapter II

THE GROWTH AND DEVELOPMENT OF COMMUNICATIVE BEHAVIOR

SENSATION AND PERCEPTUAL - MOTOR LEARNING

SENSITIVITY TO STIMULI initiates the sequence of events necessary for the development of communicative behavior. Sensitivity becomes sensation when one is aware of the stimulus and responds to it (covertly or overtly). The child's first responses are undifferentiated mass movements that are innate and reflexive. As growth and maturation occur, the child develops increasing ability to differentially respond to stimulation; that is, the child learns to recognize or perceive certain sensations and to make appropriate adjustments to them. Perceptual-motor learning is, therefore, basic to all other learning.

Because of individual differences, degree of sensitivity is an individual matter. It is quite possible, however, that certain individuals may be supersensitive because of neural lesions(4).

These people would be "more aware" of their environment. Creativity may stem from such awareness; likewise, impaired attention span, may in part, stem from such awareness.*

----

* Not much is known about creativity, i.e., is it inherited (as is commonly thought) or can it be due to some alteration of the germ plasm? We suggest another possibility, namely, that creativity might be due to the supersensitive nature of the organism caused by altered brain structure.

Similarly, impaired attention span or distractibility may stem from supersensitivity. For example, if an individual is more sensitive to his surroundings than his peer, he will be more distracted by his environment than his peer. This behavior is often exemplified in the short attention-span and distractible behavior of the brain-injured child.

Motor responses to stimulation, as previously stated, are initially undifferentiated. The growth and development of these responses proceed in an orderly, hierachical manner to discrete, differentiated responses. There are two general principles governing motor development: (1) the cephalo-caudal principle, whereby maturation proceeds from the head downwards; and (2) the proximo-distal principle, whereby maturation proceeds outwards from the axis of the body.

These principles influence the hierarchical order of differentiated motor responses. The first differentiated response will involve the head, followed by the shoulders, arms, trunk, legs, ankles, and feet. Similarly, the first reaching movements will involve gross movements of the shoulders and arms followed by more discrete movements of the hands and fingers.

If the integrity of this sequence of events is impaired, then perceptual-motor learning—our first learned behavior—is impaired. This would have significant implications for future development.

PERCEPTION

Perceptual ability develops as the child learns to recognize and discriminate his various experiences and to make the proper adjustments to these experiences. The personality structure and the motivational and attitudinal state of the growing child influence his perceptions; i.e., "he sees what he wants to see and hears what he wants to hear."

Through primitive perceptions such as movement, direction, distance, depth, size, and shape, the child begins to recognize certain relationships; that is, the child is born with the ability to "perceive" certain basic relationships but he still has to "learn" these relationships. Such learning probably takes place by virtue of trial and error, or stimulus-response type learning. The correct response to a particular stimulus rewards the organism (oftentimes it is only through trial and error behavior that the correct response is derived). The behavior is thus reinforced (strengthened) and recurs when the same stimulus is presented. Many non-human organisms develop only these primitive perceptions.

Other organisms, as does man, acquire additional perceptions based on these primitive ones by abstracting similarities into integrated perceptual wholes; e.g., letters, numbers, objects, words, etc. In such acquired perceptions, many sensory elements are usually required.

Those particular perceptual abilities which are of interest to the habilitationist are as follows:

1. *Visual Perception*
    A. Recognition-Discrimination of Space
        1) The order of letters in words
        2) The coordinates of up-down, left-right
    B. Figure-Ground Relationships
    C. Recognition-Discrimination of Distance (near-far)
    D. Recognition-Discrimination of Attributes of Form
        1) Color
        2) Size (large-small)
        3) Geometric shapes and contours
    E. Recognition-Discrimination of Form
        1) Numbers
        2) Letters
        3) Words
        4) Pictures
        5) Objects

2. *Auditory Perception*
    A. Recognition-Discrimination of the Presence of Sound
    B. Recognition-Discrimination of Wanted (speech) — Unwanted (noise) Sound, (i.e., figure-ground relationships)
    C. Recognition-Discrimination of Gross Sounds
        1) Animal sounds
        2) Musical sounds
        3) Environmental sounds (fire engine, police siren, etc.)
    D. Recognition-Discrimination of Speech Sounds
        1) Vowels
        2) Consonants

   E.   Recognition-Discrimination of the Order of Sounds in
        a Word
   F.   Recognition-Discrimination of Words
3. *Kinesthetic Perception*
   Recognition-Discrimination of body movement
4. *Tactile Perception*
   Recognition-Discrimination of Objects by Touch
5. *Integration of Perceptions*
   Similarities among the various perceptions are abstracted
   and then integrated to form new perceptions
6. *Retention of Perceptions*
   The ability to immediately recall these perceptions

CONCEPT-FORMATION

Concepts are those raw materials which, when appropriately combined, enable us to think and to fabricate judgments.

As perceptual wholes are formed by abstracting similarities from different experiences, so are concepts formed by abstracting similarities from different perceptual wholes into categories or classifications.

By category or classification, we refer to the child's ability to learn, for example, that there are different classes of animals, that there are dogs, cats, etc. It takes time, however, for the child to learn that a "big dog" and a "small dog" are still called "dogs," that there are some basic similarities that allow for this classification. Oftentimes, however, the child does not perceive these similarities and has difficulty in classifying or categorizing his experiences.

A child may incorrectly generalize his classified knowledge; for example, he might have a general concept of all adult females as being "mothers." This comes about by virtue of his own experiences with an adult female who is also his mother. Since they are one and the same, he incorrectly classifies all adult females. This, obviously, is a false generalization. Generalizations need not be false but there is always the danger that limited information will lead to false conclusions. As the child obtains more information about adult females, and about mothers, he will recognize that they may belong in different categories.

By categorizing or classifying his perceptions, the child develops an understanding of his world. It is at first a crude and basic type of understanding, but it allows him to meaningfully interact with his environment. He understands what is perceived and forms relationships between what is immediately perceived and his past perceptions, with their appropriate effects.

Lower-level abstractions, or first-learned concepts, are "concrete" because they refer or pertain to one's immediate perceptual world. As similarities are abstracted from different concepts, and as newer concepts are formed, they become more "abstract." There is a direct relationship in the degree of abstraction of a concept and in the difficulty required in learning to use it appropriately.

The term "concept," in general, has many related synonyms: idea, thought, image, and inner language.

SYMBOLIZATION

Signs, signals, codes, symbols and language are all interrelated. All are language forms, allowing for communication. All are encoded through a symbol which "refers to something" and are decoded by their respective specie, culture, or subculture. Signs and signals are codified by particular symbolic systems and each respective system may be called a language.

Our language has evolved a symbolic system of signs (V for Victory) and signals (gross sounds, e.g., siren) which are very concrete symbols. Many forms of animal life have developed this conceptual-symbolic ability. Only man, however, because of his high-level abstractions has developed a symbolic system to clothe these concepts and allow them to be communicated. Consequently we have developed words.

When there is impaired ability to understand or use the signs and signals of our language because of brain-injury the patient has an agnosia, a non-linguistic symbolization disorder. When there is difficulty in understanding and/or using our higher level symbols because of brain-injury, the patient has an aphasia, a linguistic symbolization disorder.

Language (that is, linguistic symbols) is of inestimable value to man. Through it he influences and enhances his perceptual and conceptual development and is, therefore, capable of more and more abstract thought.

It is hoped that this book, for example, through the written symbol, will help the reader to better perceive and understand the dynamics underlying communicative behavior. Likewise, the hope of every teacher is to enhance his students' ability to perceive and conceptualize the knowledge he has to impart to them.

There is a reciprocal relationship among perception, conception and language. One's perceptual and conceptual abilities influence and enhance language development; and conversely, new terminology enhances one's conceptual development.

Language Development

An enormous body of literature, relative to language development in children, has been accumulated through the years (5,8). As yet, however, there is disagreement as to how children learn language.

Myklebust has described a three stage theory that encompasses inner language, receptive language, and expressive language. Inner language might be described as that stage of language development in which the child learns to understand and manipulate his environment but does not understand the symbols representative of his environment. This understanding comes during his receptive language development; when the child understands, for example, that the word "bed" refers to the object "bed." Finally the child learns how to use these symbols in order to communicate.

It is believed that inner language is developed in the normal infant by eight or nine months, at which time he begins to develop receptive language. Expressive language, the first words uttered by the child, develops at approximately twelve or thirteen months of age.

There are disagreements in the language learning process revolving around different learning theories. The purely associationist theory, as well as the Pavlovean or Watsonian view of language learning, has been pretty well discarded. In general, reinforcement theory has supplanted these earlier ones. When responses are rewarded (or when drive-reduction occurs) the child learns; conversely, when responses are not reinforced, extinction of the behavior occurs. When a child accidentally babbles a word and is immediately rewarded by his parents with verbal or other forms of behavior, the child tends to learn this word, and he will use it again if he is desirous of obtaining a similar reward (Thorndike has labeled this the "babble-luck" theory).

Recently, Mowrer (11) has developed an autistic theory of language which suggests that the child produces many sounds or "near" words during his babbling period. When the mother produces a similar word, it gives the child a great deal of inner satisfaction and he learns to use the word. Mowrer's theory differs from the reinforcement theories, in that it rules out the babble-luck supposition of the first word.

THOUGHT

Thought may be best understood if we think of it as the "joining of ideas" springing from our concepts, and allowing for the formation of new ideas.

There are, however, three basic ways of referring to the term "thought": (1) as in the classical use of the term, whereby it refers to one's content of consciousness, e.g., "what's on your mind," or "what are you thinking about?" (2) as in problem solving, e.g., when we have to "think something out," (3) as in judgment, e.g., "do you think it's going to rain." Judgmental thinking is usually the last phase of a problem-solving episode.

Thought does not occur unless the organism is motivated to think. There are three types of motivation: (1) biological, as when we are motivated to think of food when we are hungry, etc., (2) ego-motives, such as the need for praise, self-respect, and prestige. (These derived motives are heavily influenced by the therapist, family, culture, etc.,) (3) intrinsic motives or self-motivated behavior, whereby certain stimuli are intrinsically motivating.

Chapter III

THE BRAIN MECHANISM AND
COMMUNICATIVE BEHAVIOR

THE BRAIN MECHANISM

ALL OF THE aforementioned behavior takes place because we have a brain that enables us to sense, integrate, and respond to internal and external stimuli. The brain is a complicated mechanism, and in the following pages we shall try to unveil some of its mystery.

The encephalon (brain) is composed of the following parts: cerebrum (two cerebral hemispheres covered by the cortex), brain-stem (basal-ganglia, thalamus, hypothalamus, mid-brain, pons, medulla), and cerebellum.

Cerebral Cortex

The cortex (bark) is the outer covering of the cerebrum. It is soft, spongy, and rolled up into many folds or convolutions and has seven layers of cells. In these convolutions (gyri and sulci) are found approximately fourteen billion gray cells and their underlying fibers (white substance). The cerebral cortex has been divided into four units or lobes: frontal, temporal, occipital, and parietal.

The frontal lobe, the front section of the cerebral cortex, is separated from the parietal lobe (top of head) by a deep sulcus called the fissure of Rolando, or the central sulcus. The temporal lobe, which is the lateral section of the cortex (sides of head), is separated from the frontal and parietal lobes by another deep sulcus called the lateral fissure, or the fissure of Sylvius. The

13

occipital lobe is the most caudal point of the cerebrum (back of head) and is separated from the parietal by the parietoccipital fissure.

Frontal Lobes

Immediately in front of the fissure of Rolando is the motor area for voluntary movement (area No. 4 of Brodmann). Spreading out in front of area four is another field even larger than the voluntary motor area. This nuclear field is called the pre-motor area (area No. 6). Broca's area (area No. 44) is a small area located in the posterior part of the third-left-frontal convolution, first discovered by Paul Broca in 1861 and described as a formulative and elaborative area for speech.

Patterns of motor association, engrams of words, phrases, and sentences (or our thoughts), are fed to this part of the motor cortex that controls our muscular behavior. From these areas impulses are sent to the different muscles of our body, through the descending or motor pathways, allowing for muscular activity.

Temporal Lobes

The word, "temporal" is derived from the fact that this lobe of the brain lies under the temples, at the sides of the head. "Temporal" also means "pertaining to time" and the temporal regions are very much concerned with time, time "past," as preserved in memory and time "present," as reflected in immediate retention of auditory stimuli. The lobes are also involved in a kind of false memory or false recognition called hallucinations.

Auditory stimuli are decoded in this lobe. Along the fissure of Sylvius in the superior gyrus is the primary auditory receptive area (area No. 22—Heschl's area). This site allows us to differentiate between noise and speech; that is, to recognize or perceive speech sounds. It does not, however, allow for the interpretation of these sounds. This occurs in another area (No. 41 and No. 42 — Wernicke's area) which, if damaged, results in an auditory aphasia.

Occipital Lobes

The Angular gyrus is a part of the parietal lobe that becomes continuous with the temporal and occipital lobes. It has a close relationship with the visual area (and hence is discussed under occipital lobes). Damage to the Angular gyrus results in disturbed visual-language, such as reading handicaps and writing problems.

The occipital lobe is the most caudal point of the cerebrum, and it is separated from the parietal lobe by the parieto-occipital fissure. Fibers from the optic nerve carry the retinal impressions of vision to the occipital lobe, where they are decoded.

Parietal Lobes

Into the parietal lobes, immediately behind the fissure of Rolando, come a number of sensory streams, each of which gives us information about particular aspects of our bodies: (1) tactile or touch; (2) pain; (3) temperature (different degrees of heat and different degrees of cold); (4) position sense (from proprioceptors), and (5) topognosis (an awareness of where stimuli are applied to the body).

Brain-Stem

The rest of the encephalon is called the brain-stem and is composed of a number of different parts; the striate bodies or basal ganglia (caudate, lenticular and amygdaloid nuclei; the lenticular nucleus being composed of the putamen and globis pallidus), thalamus (superior and inferior geniculate bodies), hypothalamus, mid-brain (substantia nigra, red nuclei, superior and inferior colliculi), pons, medulla, and the cerebellum (which is only connected to the brain-stem).

The basal ganglia is a collective term for a number of subcortical nuclei that at times also includes, according to different authorities, the thalamus, red nuclei, and substantia nigra. These subcortical centers cooperate with the cerebrum to control voluntary muscle movement. Phylogenetically these centers would seem to have served as motor areas but now they are primarily suppressor (restraint, or inhibitory) areas over voluntary movement. Damage to the nuclei results in a variety of different problems, according to the nucleus that is damaged. For example, athetosis, Parkinson's disease or tremors may result when one or another of these nuclei is damaged.

The thalamus probably plays some role in all of our different cortical activities. This body has ascending and descending tracts that go to and from the cortex; these pathways are sometimes called the centrencephalic system. Because of these connections, and because of its control over our emotions, the thalamus is probably responsible for the affective qualities of our different sensations. The physiological changes accompanying our emotions are mediated through the hypothalamus and its control over the autonomic nervous system which in turn, innervates and controls our physiological functions.

The mid-brain contains structures that control our sleeping and waking states, activity and rest, eating, and reproductive activities.

The pons, a body lying between the mid-brain and medulla, contains the tracts of ascending and descending fibers that connect the brain to the spinal cord. It also contains breathing centers for regulating respiratory rhythms.

The medulla lies at the bottom of the brain-stem and is in intimate contact with the spinal cord. This body also contains the ascending and descending nerve fibers, a respiratory center, cardiac center, and other vital control functions. Severe damage to this body, therefore, often results in death. The medulla, sometimes called by its full name, medulla oblongata, is also known as the bulb of the brain-stem. Bulbar paralysis, a form of polio that attacks the medulla, causes respiratory failure and almost always necessitates an "iron lung" to sustain life.

The cerebellum is connected to the brain-stem by three "arms": (1) brachia conjunctiva, that connects it to the mid-brain; (2) branchia pontis, that connects it to the pons, and (3) the restiform body, that connects it to the medulla. When cerebellar lesions are present, coordination is often impaired. Ataxia is caused by such damage.

Pyramidal System

The pyramidal system connects the sixth layer of cells in the cortico-motor area (the Betz cells—the giant pyramidal cells) with the final-common-pathway in the spinal cord. A response is organized and then sent to the motor projection areas in the frontal lobe (areas No. 4 and No. 6) and possibly to nuclei in the sub-cortex. The fibers from these nuclei carry impulses destined to control those muscles and glands engaged in the response. Some of the fibers comprising the cortico-spinal tract undoubtedly go directly from their origin in the motor and premotor areas through the brain-stem to the spinal cord. Others will synapse in the pons and medulla with the lower-motor neurons (called the cranial nerves) which lead to certain muscles. The pathway is called the corticobulbar tract (or aberrant pyramidal pathway) and it is of great importance in speech. It activates the muscles of the tongue, lips, jaw, pharynx, and larynx for the precise and purposive movements involved in speech production. If the cortical and subcortical nuclei of the pathway are injured, the nuclei of the brain-stem, having lost the control of "higher centers," will initiate characteristic activity of nonpurposive and disorganized movements. If the injury is slight, it may be noticeable only in a clumsiness of the tongue or in a tense, uninflected vocal quality.

Extrapyramidal System

Present information indicates that the extrapyramidal system is a complicated "servomechanism" for the control of the final-common-pathway. Its great importance to speech becomes apparent when we consider that it controls, activates, and inhibits the flexors and extensors, proper movement of which is necessary for coordinated activities. Damage to the extrapyramidal system is exemplified by the slow sinuous movements in athetoid type cerebral palsy where reflex tone and postures have been "freed" from control of the extrapyramidal system.

Centrencephalic System

Penfield (12) has said that integration of previous experiences takes place in a sub-cortical area; an area in which neural mechanisms are found, allowing for such integration. This system is called the centrencephalic system and is part of the reticular core.

According to Penfield, the most important part of this integration does not take place in the cerebral hemispheres. (There are, however, those who disagree with this point-of-view. It is their belief that such "business of mind" is transacted in the cerebral hemispheres by means of "association" areas in the cortex and through the transcortical fiber systems.)

It is obvious that the brain must have a central coordinating and integrating mechanism. If this "machine" is at all like other machines, there must be a place toward which streams of sensory impulses converge. There must also be a place from which streams of motor impulses emerge and are somehow summarized, making conscious planning possible.

Penfield believes that all regions of the brain may well be involved in normal conscious processes, but that the indispensable substratum of consciousness lies outside the cerebral cortex—not in the new brain but in the old, probably in the thalamus. In 1946, Penfield pointed out that Hughlings Jackson's "highest level" of integration was not located in the frontal lobes, as suggested, but in the diencephalon (thalamus and hypothalamus) and mesencephalon (midbrain). In 1952, because of criticism of the term "highest level" as suggesting separation of one level from another, the word "centrencephalic" was used to identify the integrating system.

Reticular Formation

As more research is being done on the brain, the reticular formation and centrencephalic system are receiving more and more attention. The pyramidal and extrapyramidal pathways tend to be incorporated in the reticular pathway.

This system, sometimes called a central transactional core, is neither sensory nor motor, but it affects the activity of most of the other parts of the brain. It may be subdivided into a lower and an upper system; the former being more concerned with gross excitability of muscle movement (containing facilitory and inhibitory areas), while the latter influences discrete parts of the cortex and allows for consciousness, awareness, attention, and integration to take place.

Recent studies indicate that this system exists in the central core of the brain and involves, at least, the thalamus, hypo-thalamus and midbrain. As spokes radiate from a wheel, so does the varied influence of the reticular core radiate to different parts of the brain. Some of its more important functions are as follows:

(1) It facilitates and inhibits nerve impulses.
(2) It influences incoming messages.
(3) It helps regulate glandular output through its control over the hypothalamus.
(4) It is intimately involved in perception.
(5) It affects motion.
(6) It influences wakefulness and consciousness.
(7) It allows for integration of data.

COMMUNICATIVE BEHAVIOR

There are still too many gaps in our knowledge of the brain mechanism to allow us to relate it to all kinds of communicative behavior. Questions of importance to clinicians, and relating to this topic, will be discussed:

1. *Meningitis/Encephalitis.* A careful case-history of the non-verbal child may reveal that he has suffered from meningitis or encephalitis. What do these conditions mean to the clinician? How might they be responsible for the child's non-verbalism?

The meninges envelop the cerebral cortex (which, in turn, covers the cerebral hemispheres). There are three layers of cells in the meninges: pia-mater, arachnoid, and dura-mater (the outer-most layer). Between the first two layers of cells, there is a space called the sub-arachnoid space. In the sub-arachnoid space is cerebral-spinal fluid from the ventricles, making possible a contact between the outer layers and the inner layers of the brain. (Four ventricles are in intimate contact with each other; they course throughout the brain and spinal cord, producing and containing cerebro-spinal fluid). Any infection of this fluid, therefore, may affect not only the meninges, causing meningitis (and thus cause damage to the cortex) but may also cause encephalitis, by virtue of the aforementioned contact between the ventricles and sub-arachnoid space. In encephalitis, greater damage may occur because of injury to sub-hemispherical centers. This condition is sometimes fatal.

In any case, the presence of either of these factors often reveals generalized deficiency rather than a symptom disorder.

2. *Localization vs Non-localization of Language Functions.* For the past 200 years or so, man has been critically debating this question: are there specific areas in the brain which are responsible for language formulation and its expression? The pendulum of thought has swung from those who believed in strict localization of function (that is, that many discrete parts of the brain are responsible for certain discrete communication functions), to those who believe that the brain operates as a whole. Today, most people are accepting a compromised position; that there are apparently a few large areas of the brain, rather than the whole brain, highly important for language formulation and usage. Penfield and Roberts (12) in their recent book, state that there are three areas of the brain of special significance for speech.

3. *Hemispherical Dominance and Language.* Traditionally, we believed that most right-sided individuals were left-brained (or that the left-cerebral hemisphere was dominant and vice versa). An adult who was right-sided (and most are) and who suffered damage to the left hemisphere could expect to have much difficulty in his language formulation. Such would not be the case if the damage were in the right-hemisphere. Today, however, there is a growing belief that damage to the left-hemisphere results in gross impairment to concrete language functions and that damage to the right-hemisphere results in more discrete impairment of abstract language functions. These symptoms allegedly occur regardless of sidedness (or laterality).

These symptoms may or may not be of significance regarding the non-verbal child. If a child is brain-injured in the right hemisphere, can we expect him to have difficulty understanding more abstract material as he is going into higher grades in school? Conversely, if there is an evident language problem in the young brain-injured child, can it be attributed to damage to the left hemisphere?

4. *Laterality.* During the first six years of a child's life, he alternates between hand and leg preference, gradually using one limb more than another as he grows older. By six years of age, most children consistently prefer one limb or the other. Both preferred limbs, as well as the preferred eye (and possibly ear), should be on one side of the body; that is, the child should be left-eyed, left-handed, and left-footed or vice versa. Many children, however, have "confused laterality," i.e., they prefer the left eye, right hand, and right leg, or a similar combination. Studies suggest a low but significant correlation between confused laterality and brain-injury, although we do not yet know the extent of this significance.

5. *Sensory-motor Pathways.* Sensations are brought to specific parts of the cortex (e.g., visual sensations—occipital lobe, auditory sensations—temporal lobe, sensations of touch and movement [somesthesis and kinesthesis]—parietal lobe) through affector nerves, specialized for this function. As affector nerves pass through the brain on their way to these specific sites in the cortex to be decoded, they send collaterals or branches to the reticular core. This core gathers together all previous memories concerning a particular experience.

There are three descending pathways which permit our thoughts to become responses: the pyramidal pathway transmits the impulses, the extra-pyramidal pathway coordinates the various flexor and extensor muscle groups involved in the responses, and the descending part of the reticular core controls the tone or electrical activity of the nerve response through its inhibitory and facilitory actions. Neuromotor impairment may be caused by damage to one or more of these descending pathways (cerebral palsy, for example, is a neuromotor disorder).

6. *Integration of Language Skills.* When you "think" of some person or object, you remember seeing and/or hearing and/or feeling it, etc. All of your previous experiences with the person or object are recalled and integrated into a whole. How does this process take place? Apparently our sensory memories are stored in different parts of the cortex; when the person or object is seen (or heard, or felt) or thought about, all of these previous memories are integrated, apparently through the efforts of the centrencephalic system. This system has ascending and descending fibers, connecting the various parts of the cortex to the thalamus, where integration allegedly occurs. Assuming that final integration occurs at the thalamic level of the centrencephalic system, this may also explain the presence of affective tone (or emotionality) pervading the integrated stimulus, since the thalamus is "the center of emotions." (This may explain why we sometimes react emotionally to a stranger or some experience —because of past experience with a person resembling the stranger, etc.)

7. *Emotionality.* Oftentimes the clinician finds himself working with (or examining) a child who is hyper-emotional, or whose case-history indicates hyper-emotionality, such as excessive or uncontrollable crying or laughing, fear or anger, etc. Such conditions are oftentimes part of a syndrome that accompanies non-verbalism and is symptomatic of pathology to the thalamus.

8. *Neuromuscular Pathology.* Any damage to the cortex and subcortical areas (including the brain-stem and cerebellum) may result in impaired articulation (dysarthria), voice, rhythm, or language. It is only when there is cortical pathology, however, that language disorders may appear (excluding those caused by hearing loss); conversely, insult to any other part of the brain may result in any one or more of the other speech disorders. These disorders are characterized by the following abnormal neuro-muscular conditions:

1. Impaired sequential movement—Apraxia
2. Incoordination—Ataxia
3. Rigid muscles—Rigidity
4. Writhing muscles—Athetosis
5. Impaired tonus—Paralysis or Paresis
6. Tremorous muscles—Tremor

A. *Impaired Sequential Movement (Apraxia).* The kinesthetic memory for sequential behavior is impaired in this disorder, and is characterized by clumsiness and/or awkwardness. Many young children who are awkward may be suffering from a form of this disorder which makes sequential learning difficult.

B. *Incoordination (Ataxia).* As one talks, the jaw is opening and closing, requiring flexor and extensor movement (agonist/antagonist) of the muscles involved in jaw movement. These opposing muscle movements must be completely coordinated if smooth muscular responses are to occur. A flexor (or extensor) muscle group sends a constant stream of information regarding its movements to the cerebellum through proprioceptors, the specialized receptors for movement. The cerebellum, in turn, sends information to the opposing muscle and allows for the constancy of the flexion and extension. Such normal movements are called synergic movements; whereas disordered functioning is asynergic and results in ataxia.

C. *Rigid Muscles (Rigidity)*. This condition is caused by marked increase in muscle tone and is usually characterized by a "lead-pipe type paralysis."

D. *Writhing Muscles (Athetosis)*. Athetosis is caused by damage to certain nuclei of the extra-pyramidal system which normally suppress the purposeless, slow, writhing movements characteristic of this disorder. When these nuclei are damaged, the suppression is lifted resulting in the release of this primitive automatism.

E. *Impaired Tonus (Paralysis or Paresis)*. Neural tone, or the constant stream of neural activity (or excitability), may become hypertonic or hypotonic (resulting in spastic or flaccid muscles) due to injury to various parts of the brain. Apparently there are certain areas of the brain which control and regulate neural tone, namely, the suppressor and facilitory areas. Damage to the former means that normal suppression (or restraint or inhibition) cannot be applied to the nerve impulse, and as a result the muscle(s) it feeds becomes spastic; conversely, when there isn't proper facilitation, the muscle(s) becomes flaccid. Whenever there is impaired tonus, the affected muscles become paralyzed or paretic (semi-paralysis).

F. *Tremorous Muscles (Tremors)*. Tremors are caused by improper distribution of tone to the muscles, usually because of damage to the Basal Ganglia. There are resting and intention tremors; in the former they are only apparent when the patient is at rest, and the latter appear only when he is engaged in some activity.

A disease such as Saint Vitus Dance (Chorea) causes choreiform movements to appear which are quite similar to the abovementioned tremors. Parkinson's disease causes both resting tremors and rigidity. Paralysis agitans, or "shaking palsy" is manifested by resting tremors.

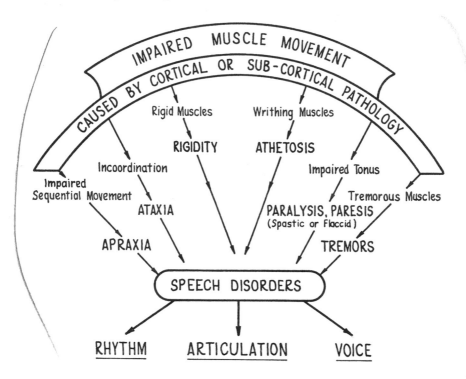

9. *Sensory-motor Servomechanism.* All responses are fed back into our computer-type brain and scanned, analyzed, and compared to previously learned standards. If a discrepancy is noted between the present and previously learned standard of behavior, then an immediate rectification is made. This "feeding back" of information (or automatic self-regulation) is best exemplified in the hearing mechanism. Our ability to hear ourselves as we talk (side-tone), thereby monitoring our voices or articulation, is an example of an automatic servomechanism.

10.   *The Brain and Intelligence.* As stated elsewhere in this book, intelligence is a compound of many facets and is related, in part, to the integrity of brain structure and functioning. All causes of mental subnormality are directly related to either impaired structure (mal-development or brain-injury) or functioning or both. In this way, we can say that any non-verbal child is also a mentally subnormal child, since language development is a facet of intelligence. We can carry this discussion even farther afield by saying that all causes of non-verbalism are, therefore, related to alterations of brain structure or functioning or both; thus, the emotionally ill child with a concomitant language problem has disturbed functioning of his brain.

Chapter IV

SYMPTOMS OF DYSFUNCTION

W<small>HEN A THERAPIST</small> is examining or working with a child who is significantly delayed in his language development, he should be aware of other possible problems which may exist. In this chapter, we intend to explore other significant and accompanying symptoms.

AUDITORY*

Hearing and speech are intimately related. If speech is present, we know that the child at least hears the spoken word or that deafness (or severe hearing loss) occured after speech was acquired. The very young deaf child does not vocalize for pleasure as much as he uses his voice to call attention to his needs. Since he does not hear his own voice, it has a characteristic non-melodious quality typical of the deaf child. He can, however, use and understand gestures. The deaf child might make more use of his senses and acquire more sensitivity, for example, to visual clues and tactile sensations (re: vibrations) because of his lack of auditory sensitivity. The motor development of the deaf child is normal for his age, which is in contrast to the brain-damaged and mentally deficient child. The deaf child's gait may be peculiar, however, in that he may shuffle and drag his feet while walking. This might be due to the fact that

----

* We have deliberately omitted visual dysfunctions. However, the reader should, of course, be aware that such dysfunction does occur.

he does not hear himself walking. Vestibular function may also be deficient, and poor balance may be observed.

Inconsistent auditory dysfunction is sometimes found as a concomitant of non-verbalism. This disorder, called by a variety of names (auditory imperception, auditory aphasia, etc.), is symptomatic of cortical brain-injury. This type of child can hear well, but he has difficulty in decoding the auditory message whether it be a linguistic or non-linguistic symbol, and hence he oftentimes tends to "tune-out" to auditory stimuli. This inconsistent "tuning-out" causes his auditory behavior to be somewhat characteristic of the negativistic child (children between two and five years of age make much use of this technique to manipulate their environment) and is oftentimes confused with it.

PERCEPTUAL

There are many possible symptoms of perceptual impairment ranging from the discrete, localized problem to the all-inclusive perceptual disorder. These symptoms are as follows:

1. **Visual Dysfunction**

   (a) Impaired recognition of the order of letters in words, characterized by impaired reading and writing ability. In reading, the child is likely to misread words, or say words backwards as "nip" instead of "pin." In writing he is likely to write words incorrectly or write words backwards, as in the above example.

   (b) Impaired recognition of visual coordinates, i.e., up-down, left-right. When reading he may read from right to left or down and up. His writing may be characterized by a similar disorder.

   (c) Impaired recognition of foreground when it is against a background, characterized by slow reading, impaired ability to work a puzzle, etc.

   (d) Impaired recognition of distance, as manifested in writing disturbances in which the child has difficulty in writing on a line, or spacing his words to prevent "cramping," or coloring within a limited boundary. He might also confuse near and far relationships and judge distances incorrectly, as when throwing something at an object. When reading, he might hold the book very close to his face.

(e) Impaired recognition of color, size, or shape, as manifested in faulty recognition of objects, pictures, numbers, letters, and words. This disorder might be manifested in reading problems, in which the child confuses certain letters or words, or in writing disturbances.

Lehtinen (7) has succinctly described the perceptual problem as follows:

a. *Visual Perception*

Our tests are not yet adequate to isolate and describe these deficits with precision, but with some of them we can come rather close. It is useful to know what the child's visual perceptual functioning is like—how well he can discriminate forms, organize the space of a page, hold a figure against a disturbing background, see relationships among several elements presented at one time, analyze a figure into its parts and recombine them, and handle without confusion the coordinates of up-down, right and left.

A deficit in the abilities usually reflects directly in the child's school and play performances. In learning to read, the child confuses m, n, e, c, h, n, y, and v because his form discrimination is inaccurate. He confuses p, d, b, m. and w because his spatial orientation is unstable. In writing he is likely to reverse numbers and letters. In number work he counts inaccurately and forgets where he began because he has difficulty holding the separate parts of a number grouping in a stable pattern. In drawing he produces unrecognizable forms or distorts even simple patterns like a triangle or a diamond. In play, the child with these visual perceptual problems is unsuccessful with puzzles, in playing checkers, in block building, in tinker toy construction and so on because these involve perceiving the relationship of parts to one another in order to form a whole.

b. *Auditory Perception*

The level and quality of the child's auditory perceptual organization is of interest to us too. This includes a knowledge of whether he can discriminate sounds which are quite similar as i and e, sh and ch, and so on, whether he can combine or blend syllables or separate sounds into a word, whether he can detect similarities in the sounds of words—either the beginning or ending or vowel sounds, and whether he can analyze a word sound into its several parts. Difficulties in auditory perception are usually reflected in a child's speech. To such a child "milk" and "melk"; or "Indian" and "Endian" are not different. Rather than hearing "put the ball away," he may hear "pit the ball away." "Chicken" may be pronounced "shicken." This child will almost certainly have difficulty in reading—if not in the first grade, later when he must read independently. A child with difficulties in synthesizing two sounds may know the separate sounds but repeat them over and over—being quite unable to "hear" or perceive them as a single word. A child with difficulty in analyzing a word into its parts perceives the meaning of a word rather than its sounds. "Danny" is a boy's name but not the combination of two sound units "Dan," "ny."

CONCEPTUAL

Conceptual dysfunction is characterized by concretized thought and a paucity of ideas. The patient is unable to understand or use abstractions of varying difficulty, so that he may resort to gestures or emotional evocations to express himself. School subjects, such as spelling or arithmetic, will offer little difficulty. More abstract subjects, such as reading and others in the language arts, will present greater difficulty.

LANGUAGE

The child seems to be unable to understand or use nonlinguistic language and/or linguistic language symbols appropriate to his age.

THOUGHT

Impaired thinking ability may be manifested by any of a number of disorders:

1. *Impairment in the Progression of Thought*
   a. Impaired spontaneity of thought.
   b. Retardation of ideas or a poverty of expression of ideas.

    c. Perseveration or the persistent repetition of the same response regardless of the flow of thought.

    d. Blocking or obstruction of the flow of thought.

    e. Flight of ideas or the rapid succession of ideas basically unrelated to each other.

    f. Incoherence or the disorderly progression of ideas.

2. *Impairment of the Form of Thought*

    a. Echolalia or the persistent and meaningless repetition of another's words.

    b. Neologisms or the coining of meaningless words.

    c. Word salad or a jumble of meaningless words.

3. *Impairment of the Content of Thought*

    a. Fantasy (autistic) or the morbid egocentric distortion of thought (wishfulfilling).

    b. Obsession or a persistent symbolic thought.

    c. Fixed idea or a persistent idea out of logical context.

MOTOR (CEREBRAL PALSY)

When brain-injury in a child (before, during, or after birth) causes improper neural control over muscular behavior, and hence improper muscular movement, we may say that the child has cerebral palsy. Damage to a specific area of the brain usually results in characteristic observable signs, e.g., a lesion in the basal ganglia may result in athetosis, a lesion in the motor cortex may result in spasticity, and damage to the cerebellum may result in ataxia, etc.

There are five main types of cerebral palsy: spastic, athetoid, rigidity, ataxic, and tremors. Occasionally, mixed types occur.

1. *Spastic Type.* A spastic child is identified by stiffness. His motions are accurate, but he makes them slowly and with great effort. He moves slowly and only a little at a time. He may be unable to enunciate properly or to use words and sentences. When he attempts to bend a joint, the opposing muscles may contract and trigger off the stretch reflex.

There are more children with this type of cerebral palsy than any other type: in spastic quadriplegia, the child's arms and legs are both involved; when the lower half of the body is involved, a child is described as having paraplegia; a third sub-group is characterized by hemiplegia where one side of the body is affected, the other side being normal; diplegia is paralysis of either both arms or both legs.

Spasticity may be defined as an impairment of muscle tone due to simultaneous contraction of antagonistic or reciprocal muscle groups (flexors and extensors) accompanied by a definite degree of hypertension or hypertonicity.

2. *Athetoid Type.* Athetosis is the second most common type of cerebral palsy. Athetoids are constantly in motion. The child moves when he does not want to move; he has difficulty in controlling his arms, legs, and/or speech muscles. These involuntary motions are clearly different from the stiffness which characterizes the spastic child. In the arm, they are especially noticeable when a child attempts to write or hold a glass of water, toy, or other object. When the effort to counteract this excess motion becomes habitual, the resulting counter-contraction of the muscles produces a different syndrome called "tension athetosis," which is similar to spasticity. The athetoids' movements are absent during sleep.

There is general agreement that athetosis is the result of a lesion of the extra-pyramidal system, but all the areas and tracts comprising this system still are undetermined. Some authorities would limit the lesion to the basal nuclei (striate bodies) and the pathways proceeding to and from these nuclei. One may conclude that the site and degree of damage to the extra-pyramidal system will determine the specific characteristic of the motor behavior of the athetoid. There are various types of athetosis. They range from the extremely mild cases to the serious ones involving rapid and constant involuntary motions.

3. *Rigidity Type.* Children in this group are slow-moving. They have difficulty in extending their arms and legs fully because their muscles are partially contracted all of the time. They are rigid at certain times, but at other times they can move about with comparative freedom. The aim of treatment in this group is to speed up motion and to improve balance and control of the arms, legs, and tongue.

The rigidity is due to a combined resistance of agonist and antagonist muscles. Most of these children are mentally defective.

4. *Ataxic Type.* Ataxic children are incoordinate and have a poor sense of balance. Damage to the cerebellum interferes with the feeding-back of information to the flexor and extensor muscle groups resulting in asynergic or incoordinated movements.

5. *Tremor Type.* This is the least frequent type of cerebral palsy. It is often referred to as the shaking palsy. The hands, arms, or neck shake back and forth in a rhythmical manner. Tremors are apparent as soon as the child is old enough to use his arms or legs in any way.

Chapter V

TESTING FOR THE VARIOUS DYSFUNCTIONS

INTRODUCTION

T HERE IS NEED for a comprehensive test that will examine all of the events previously discussed; the results of which will be clinically useful in the habilitation program for the young child. This chapter makes an attempt to fulfill this need.

Giving a test and scoring errors is simply not enough, however. One must be able to interpret the results and clinically use the information thus obtained.

The examiner, of course, wants to determine what functions are defective; but just as important (if not more so) is to determine whether or not these defective functions are secondary to some other disturbance. For example, if you hold a pencil before a patient and ask, "What is this?" you have to determine by his response, and his other responses, wherein the difficulty lies. It isn't enough to know that the patient could not identify the object. Is his inability, for example, related to: (1) an inability to *attend* to the stimulus for a sufficient length of time? (2) an inability to *remember its name* although he can describe its use. (3) an inability to *recognize* the *object*. (4) an inability to *recognize* the object because of *impaired visual form, shape, or size perception*. (5) an inability to *recognize* the object because of *auditory impairment*: hearing loss, short auditory retention span, or impaired auditory perception of various types (difficulty in discriminating speech from noise, difficulty in discrimination of various speech sounds, etc.). (6) an inability to say the *word*, or say it correctly, because of *disturbed functioning* of the speech mechanism.

This talent, the examiner's ability to differentially diagnose, comes with experience.

AUDITORY

In order to rule out the possibility of deafness, one must get some idea of the child's auditory acuity. Auditory tests for young children may be classified as formal and informal. The formal tests include pure-tone audiometry, tuning forks, and speech audiometry, all of which require active cooperation on the part of the child. Another formal but more objective test is Electrodermal Audiometry (E.D.R.), otherwise known as Psychogalvanometry (P.G.S.R.). Informal tests do not require active cooperation and they include sound instruments, sound toys, and free field noise and voice tests.

Due to immaturity and/or dysfunction, the child will often have to be tested informally. A test that may be appropriately used is the "sound instrument test." The child is seated and encouraged to play with a toy while the examiner produces a sound from a musical instrument (or noise-maker) that is not visible to the child. The examiner watches for any reaction. Another informal test is the "sound toy test," especially useful in diagnosing emotionally disturbed children who do not respond to sound. The child is given a toy that produces a sound not louder than conversational speech, such as a doll or telephone, and he is encouraged to play with it. If a sound occurs unintentionally and the child hears it, there may be some visible reaction. If the child then produces the sound again, intentionally, it is another indication that he hears. This test is particularly useful with the autistic child who apparently rejects sounds from his environment but who often accepts sound that he himself produces. Some children who do not respond to sound will respond to the *absence* of sound, i.e., when given two toys, one of which does not produce sound, they will detect the difference between them. Free field tests are the preferred tests and may employ social sounds with which the child is familiar, or pure-tone or noise stimuli at various intensities (this test necessitates a sound-proof, two room test chamber). The examiner watches for responses or reaction to these sounds. Usually one can get an idea of the child's auditory acuity by the use of these tests. If there is any suggestion of hearing loss, the child should then be referred to a qualified audiologist for a further and more comprehensive test.

PERCEPTUAL

1. The following is suggested for **visual dysfunction:**
   A. *Space Perception*
      1. Have the patient read a simple passage (if capable of reading).
         a. Does he reverse words?
         b. Does he read from the wrong coordinate (right to left)?
         c. Is he a poor reader?
      2. Have the patient write a few simple words, e.g., man, etc. (if capable of writing words).
         a. Does he spell the words incorrectly?
         b. Does he reverse words (e.g., god instead of dog)?
         c. Are letters incorrectly juxtaposed?
         d. Does he write from the wrong coordinate?
   B. *Figure-ground Disturbance*
      1. Does he misread words, numbers, letters, or detect incorrect figures when presented on a checkered or on different colored backgrounds?
      2. Is he unsuccessful in manipulating simple puzzles? (If so, examiner must first rule out perceptual motor or any eye-hand coordination difficulty before deciding on figure-ground as the factor.)
   C. *Distance Perception*
      1. Have the patient write a sentence.
         a. Does his writing not come close to the line?
         b. Are his words cramped together?
      2. Have the patient color within a circle.
         a. Does color extend over line?
         b. Does color not come close to line?

3. Have the patient throw an object at another object.
    a. Does he completely overshoot his mark?
    b. Does he completely undershoot his mark?

D. *Shape (contour), Size, and Color Perception*
    1. Shape—Present two sets of cards of varying shapes
       and have the patient make appropriate matches.
    2. Size—The tester should present several different
       sized objects before the child. The child is in-
       structed to show the one that is the largest, smallest,
       next largest, etc. The tester can then have the
       child attempt to put the objects in order, ranging
       from largest to smallest or from smallest to largest.
       A recommended testing implement is a color cone,
       the parts of which range in size from small to
       large or vice versa in sequential order.
    3. Colors—The tester should show the child swatches
       of material (felt material is recommended since it
       can be used on a flannel board) and indicate to him
       that he is to match the colors with a duplicate set
       of colored swatches; or the previously mentioned
       color cone can be used. If the child can match
       colors of *identical* items, test his ability to match
       colors of *dissimilar* items (thereby ruling out the
       possibility of shape and size cues as visual aids to
       discrimination.) He can, for instance, be instructed
       to match a piece of the material to its corresponding
       color on the color cone.

E. *Form Perception*
    1. The tester should have the child match a series of
       small wooden blocks in the forms of a circle, a cross,
       a triangle, and a square. A simple puzzle is also
       good for testing the child's ability to perceive visual
       form as well as visual size and orientation in space.
    2. Have duplicates of letters, words, and numbers and
       have patient make appropriate matches.
        a. Letters—In this area, the tester should observe
           whether or not the child can match the letters

of the alphabet (an "A" with an "A" etc.). The letters should be presented in both printed and cursive style in order to check for an ability to recognize one but not the other.

b. Words—The tester should check for whether or not the child can recognize simple words such as pig, puppy, pie, cat, etc. If the child cannot speak or indicate in such a way that he knows the word, present him with a duplicate set of words being used and observe whether or not he can match the words correctly.

c. Numbers—The tester should have a duplicate set of number cards. If the child cannot indicate orally the recognition of a number or numbers, he should be given the opportunity to match like numbers. If the child cannot recognize numbers, it would seem almost certain that he would be deficient in calculation ability (arithmetic) also. However, if the child does recognize numbers, tests for mathematical ability can also be administered. The tester can present the child with cards that involve simple mathematical problems (2—2=?) and with other cards of individual numbers. The child is to look at the problem and then pick out the appropriate answer from among the individual number cards.

2. The following is suggested for **auditory dysfunction:**

A. *Presence or absence of sound*—The tester should be looking for the ability or inability of the child to recognize and discriminate the presence of sound. The examiner should first check to see if there is any response to sound by clapping his hands behind the child's back and noticing whether or not the child responds to the sound or looks for the sound source (accurately or inaccurately).

B. *Gross sounds*—In testing for the recognition and discrimination of gross sounds, the examiner should determine whether the child recognizes environmental sounds, animal sounds, musical sounds, etc. With a selection of sound-producing objects placed on the examining table, the tester should produce a sound, when the childs eyes are closed, and have the child indicate which object made the noise.

C. *Speech sounds*—The examiner can determine whether or not the child can discriminate among different sounds by having him indicate or raise his hand when he hears "his" sound.

The recognition and discrimination of words can be tested by instructing the child to point to objects in the room, parts of the body, etc. For example, the examiner can ask the child, "Do you have a nose?" If the child responds in the affirmative, the examiner can ask, "Where is it?" The examiner can also present identical or different "word pairs" and ask the child to indicate if they were the same or different.

3. The following is suggested for **tactile dysfunction:**

Tests in this area might first include having the child "feel" certain objects while blindfolded or while his eyes are closed. He is then instructed to open his eyes and identify the object he felt from a group of several objects placed in front of him. Next, the child might be instructed to close his eyes while the examiner touches certain parts of the body (eyes, ears, arm). The child then indicates what part of the body was touched.

The examiner should administer the tests so that he will discover any indication of unilateral or bilateral tactile dysfunction. He should have the child feel the objects with each hand individually and with both hands simultaneously.

4. The following is suggested for **kinesthetic dysfunction:**

Take the patient's hand and, with his eyes closed, make a number or letter in the air. Can the child identify or match the movement involved?

5. The following is suggested for **visual retention dysfunction:**

Point to a series of objects (pictures will do), asking the patient to repeat the performance in the exact order. Compare his performance to a peer group. Is there a difference in ability? (When giving directions for test, keep verbal explanation to a minimum in case the patient has a reduced auditory retention span. Use pantomime as much as possible.)

6. The following is suggested for **auditory retention dysfunction:**

   Ask the patient to repeat numbers, e.g., 2-5, 3-7-1, etc. (Using a monotone voice, space each number presentation by a one-second pause.)

   The norms are as follows:

Age	Number of Digits
3	3
4	4
7	5
10	6
14	7
18	8

7. The following is suggested for testing **body-image:**

   A. For visual dysfunction the following procedures can be used:
      1. "Do you have legs?" "Show me the right one."
      2. "Show me your left hand."
      3. "Put the bracelet on your left arm."

   It is important to remember that auditory recognition, retention, and visual distance abilities are involved in the correct response to this test; e.g., if the patient has difficulty in recognizing or retaining the auditory command, he will not be able to respond appropriately; likewise a difficulty in perceiving visual distance can cause the patient to "overshoot" or "undershoot" the mark, leaving the impression that he had distorted body image.

   B. The examiner should test for general understanding of the "parts" relationship of many "bodies" by having the child draw a man, a dog, a tree, and a house. *The examiner is looking for incorrect and distorted recognition of the relationship of the parts that go together.* The examiner should always be watching for any clues to other types of disorders that might manifest themselves during the testing procedure.

CONCEPTUAL

The examiner should be concerned with the child's ability to categorize or classify stimuli. To this end the following ideas can be used to test the child:

1. *Classification of likeness*:
   Present a variety of different stimuli and ask the child to put those that are similar in separate bundles.
2. *Discrimination of differences*:
   Present visual and auditory stimuli; in the former the pictures should be incomplete; in the latter the sounds should be dissimilar.
   a. visual differences—what is missing
   b. auditory differences—how is it different
3. *Classifications*:
   Ask the child what the following stimuli are called:
   a. dog, cat, horse, cow (animals)
   b. peach, grapes, banana (fruit)
   c. chair, sofa, table (furniture)
4. *More abstract concepts*:
   a. holidays—present a picture and ask what and why, etc.
   b. seasons of year—present a picture and ask when, what to wear, etc.
   c. sequential order—tell a story and ask what happened, when, etc.

LANGUAGE

1. There are four facets of language development that should be tested:

   a. *Inner language development*—give the patient certain items, e.g., wearing apparel, toy house furniture, etc.

Does he know their proper uses, appropriate place-
ments, etc.?

b. *Receptive language development*
c. *Expressive language development*
d. *Connected speech development*

Receptive language can be tested by using either the Full-
Range Picture Vocabulary Test or the Peabody Picture Vocabulary Test.* Expressive language can be determined by comparing the patient's ability to name objects according to the
Lerea and/or Freeman Norms. Similarly, connected speech
development or the number of words used in a sentence, can be
determined by comparing the child's responses to the McCarthy
Norms. More specific language tests are as follows:

The Lerea-Freeman Norms and the McCarthy Norms are as follows:

Words	Lerea's	Freeman's
fire	3 years	3 years
rake	3 years	3 years
toe	3 years	4 years
owl	4 years	4 years
spider	4 years	4 years
church	4 years	5 years
rainbow	5 years	5 years
horseshoe	5 years	5 years
arrow	5 years	7 years
apron	6 years	4 years
bench	5 years	5 years
lock	6 years	6 years
faucet	7 years	7 years
vase	7 years	6 years
grave	8 years	7 years
cuff	8 years	8 years
jar	8 years	7 years

---

* The Full-Range Picture Vocabulary Test can be obtained from the
Psychological Test Specialists, Box 1441, Missoula, Montana. The Peabody
Picture Vocabulary Test can be obtained from the American Guidance Service,
Inc., 2106 Pierce Avenue, Nashville 12, Tennessee.

McCarthy Norms

Age	Number of Words/Sentences
1.5	1
2.5	2
3.5	3
4.5	4
5.5	5
6.5	6
7.5	7
8.5	7
9.5	7

The following developmental schedule will also be of use to the clinician in evaluating and enhancing language skills. For a more complete and detailed discussion the reader is referred to M. J. Mecham's "Verbal Language Development Scale," Springfield Illinois. Educational Test Bureau, or by the same author, "Developmental Schedules of Oral-Aural Language As An Aid to the Teacher of the Mentally Retarded," *Mentally Retarded*, December, 1963.

	Language Skill	In Descending Order of Difficulty	Approximate Age
1.	Follow simple instructions		1 -
2.	Recognizes names of most common objects		
3.	Recognizes parts of the body when they are named.		
4.	Expressive vocabulary of 10 or more words		1 - 5
5.	Identifies common pictures when they are named		
6.	Talks in short sentences		
7.	Names a few common pictures		2 -
4.	Expressive vocabulary of at least 50 words		1.5
9.	Uses pronouns, such as I, me, you, etc.		2.5
10.	Recognizes action in pictures		
11.	Names one color		
12.	Auditory memory span of two words		3 -
13.	Understands prepositions such as over, under, above, on, etc.		
14.	Has mastered the p, b, m, h, and w sounds		3.5

15. Says at least one nursery rhyme or poem or sings a simple song or two with most of the essential detail
16. Auditory memory span of four words   4 -
17. Names all primary colors
18. Reads aloud by way of pictures   4.5
19. Mastery of y (j), k, g, v, t, d
20. Expresses himself in dramatic play activities   5 -

2. The diagnosis of Non-Linguistic Symbolization Impairments
   A. *Visual*
      1. Present visual signs and have patient indicate in some way (if possible have objects the signs represent) that he understands its meaning, e.g., plus and minus signs, dollar signs, etc.
   B. *Auditory*
      Present recordings of gross sounds (e.g., animal sounds, environmental sounds) and ask patient to identify them by relating them to the appropriate object or picture. Does he understand the relationship between the sound and that which it represents? This is unlike auditory perception where only recognition and discrimination are involved and not meaning.
   C. *Tactile*
      Place different objects in his hand and ask him what they are *for* (eyes closed) e.g., pencil, key, coin, comb, etc.

3. The diagnosis of Linguistic Symbolization Disorders
   1. *Receptive Disorders*
      a. *Visual*—If the patient can read, start with simple sentences. Progress to short stories. Have the child read the material silently and answer written questions pertaining to the material with a yes or no response.
      b. *Auditory*
         1. Present commands ranging from simple to com-

plex that do not involve a verbal response, e.g., open the book, close the book, stand up, go to the window, point to the......., etc.
2. Read a simple story to the child and ask questions concerning its content.
3. Present correct and incorrect statements to the child and ask for his responses, e.g., I have two heads—yes or no.

2. *Expressive Disorders*
   a. *Verbal Language*
     1. Naming ability—have child name objects or pictures, e.g., pencil, key, coin, comb, etc. by asking, "What is this called?" (See test for expressive language development.)
     2. Word finding ability—ask child simple questions, e.g., "What do you sleep in?" "What day is today?" "What was yesterday?" "What are a dog, a cat, and a horse called?" etc.
     3. *Functional speech*—if the child has the mental ability, ask him to define or explain certain words, e.g., "What does 'apple' mean?" (Keep the words concrete.)
   b. *Writing*
     Present simple words for the patient to write; e.g., cat, dog, horse, etc. Does he write the wrong word? We are not concerned here with *how* he writes the word as long as he can write the correct word (spelling errors may or may not be significant).

NEUROMOTOR

When testing the speech mechanism for symptoms of neuromotor impairment the following procedures can be followed:
1. *Respiration*—can the child sustain a continuous expiration of air for at least ten seconds?
2. *Phonation*—can the child sustain a continuous phonation of *ah* for at least ten seconds?

3. *Resonation*—examine the velopharyngeal structure (soft-palate and pharyngeal wall) as the child phonates for brief periods the *ah* sound. Does the soft palate elevate and go straight back each time? Look for a partial paralysis (paresis) by carefully noticing if the velopharyngeal activity is normal during each phonation of the *ah*. Does the uvula and/or soft palate deviate to one side? If so, this may indicate the presence of an unilateral paralysis.

4. *Articulation*—check tongue movements. Is there any impairment of muscle tone as characterized by flaccidity or spasticity? Is muscle movement slow or sluggish? Look for ataxic or apraxic tongue movements by having the patient touch a tongue depressor placed along the sides of his lips with his tongue. If tongue movements are awkward and he is unable to touch the depressor, have him look into a mirror as he repeats the task. Is he better? If so, this might suggest an apraxic tongue. If not, it may be an ataxic tongue (but first rule-out other possible causes of incorrect tongue movements such as tongue-tie, "lazy" tongues, etc.). Another test is to ask the patient to touch certain parts of the palate or mouth after you previously touched them. Can he locate the exact spot?
One can test lip action by having the patient smile; do the lips spread evenly or is there distortion?
Jaw movements can be tested by simply having the patient open and close his mouth as rapidly as possible. Does this activity appear normal?

A gross neurological examination can also be performed by the therapist. The following would comprise this examination (some of these techniques would be difficult to use with a young child).

1. The examination really starts when the patient (client) enters and the examiner sees him walking. The examiner notices, generally, the posture and any unusual manner of carrying the head, arms, or legs. Specifically, gait should be checked.

2. *Atrophy of body*—the examiner can notice any wasting of the arms or legs, flaccid paralysis, or rigidity of visible body parts.

3. *Hand tremors*—have the individual extend arms parallel, shoulder high to the front of the body with palms down. Place a sheet of paper across both hands. Tremors are suggestive of lesions of the basal ganglia.
Have the individual extend arms horizontally to the sides. With eyes open or closed, tell him to touch the tip of the nose with the index finger, using each hand in turn. Over- or-under shooting is suggestive of cerebellar damage . . . this is the so-called dysmetria effect. This can be further checked by asking the individual to bring the heel of one foot to the knee of the other leg, and vice versa. In other words, dysnynergic action leads to misdirection.

4. *Rebound phenomenon* (disturbance in synergic balance in the muscles of motor unit). When the examiner taps a stiffened, outstretched arm in a downward direction, his response is normal if there is little upward movement. In cerebellar disease, the limb rebounds with an upward fling which exceeds the normal excursion because the antagonists fail to exert the normal check.

5. *Adiadochokinesis*—the name applied to a slow, irregular clumsiness elicited in quick alternating movements such as supination to pronation in the upper limbs. This may be tested by seating the client with legs together with feet flat on floor and then asking him rapidly to tap the knees with the palms and then the backs of the hands. Again, this is suggestive of cerebellar defects.

6. *Romberg's test*—have the client stand (preferably with shoes off) with heels and toes together, eyes closed. Considerable sway is a positive sign of cerebellar defect. Test can be made more sensitive by having client stand on one foot (eyes still closed) and then on the other. (Examiner should stand close by to catch client if he starts to fall. The ability to see causes the disappearance of this form of ataxia and reappears when the eyes are shut.)

7. *Tabes Dorsalis* (syphilis of C.N.S.)—can be suspected if client walks with broadbased gait which becomes noticeably worse when eyes are closed. If the gait does not become worse when eyes are closed, other forms of cerebral damage might be suggested.

8. *Testing grip*—have patient squeeze examiner's hand.

9. *Thumb-finger opposition*—have the individual tap thumb with each finger of the same hand (test both hands separately) rapidly and accurately. A poor performance may be due to faulty synergy and lowered tonus, suggestive of neocerebellar disease.

10. *Finger-to-finger test*—have patient extend index fingers to examiner's index fingers—have him close his eyes and withdraw his fingers—then try to extend index fingers and touch index fingers of examiner again. Great deviation on either side is suggestive of cortical lesion on the opposite side.

SPECIFIC NEUROLOGICAL EXAMINATIONS— CRANIAL NERVES

Number of Nerve:	I.
Name of Nerve:	Olfactory
Origin in Brain:	Ventral parts of cerebral hemisphere
Function:	Smell (sensory)
Neurological Test:	Use some non-irritating substance such as cloves, coffee, etc. Have client shut off one nostril and sniff with other—do each in turn.
Number of Nerve:	II.
Name of Nerve:	Optic
Origin in Brain:	Thalamus
Function:	Vision (sensory)
Neurological Test:	Close each eye in turn—hold up varying number of fingers to open eye, moving fingers from edge to center to edge.
Number of Nerve:	III.
Name of Nerve:	Occulomotor
Origin in Brain:	Midbrain
Function:	Eye movement (motor)
Neurological Test:	(1) Contraction with approach of bright light to eye. (2) Accommodation—examiner extends finger toward client's nose—if normal, eyes should contract or narrow.

(3) Hold lids open—tilt head back—eyeballs should go up.

(4) Pursuit movement—hold head in fixed position straight ahead and have client follow—with his eyes—movement of examiner's finger from edge to center—can be checked at the same time as testing optic nerve.

Number of Nerve:	IV.
Name of Nerve:	Trochlear
Origin in Brain:	Midbrain
Function:	Eye movement (motor)
Neurological Test:	Same test as for III.

Number of Nerve:	VI.°
Name of Nerve:	Abducens
Origin in Brain:	Medulla
Function:	Eye movement (motor)
Neurological Test:	Same test as for III and IV.

Number of Nerve:	V.
Name of Nerve:	Trigeminal
Origin in Brain:	Midbrain and Pons
Function:	Masticatory movement (motor)
Neurological Test:	(1) Jaw jerk
	(2) Place hands along client's jaw (examiner stands in back)—have client grind teeth together. If normal there should be smooth strong feel of jaw muscles.

Number of Nerve:	VII.
Name of Nerve:	Facial
Origin in Brain:	Medulla
Function:	Facial movement (motor)
Neurological Test:	Check muscles of expression by asking patient to smile.

Number of Nerve:	VIII.
Name of Nerve:	Auditory vestibular
Origin in Brain:	Medulla
Function:	Hearing (sensory)
Neurological Test:	Test hearing by previously mentioned techniques.

Number of Nerve:	IX.
Name of Nerve:	Glossopharyngeal
Origin in Brain:	Medulla
Function:	Tongue (sensory) Pharynx (motor)
Neurological Test:	Have client swallow. If uvula goes straight up—normal. If it deviates to either side—suggestive of paralysis on opposite side.

° Note change in numerical order done to group together nerves III, IV and VI (concerned with eye movements).

Number of Nerve:	X.
Name of Nerve:	Vagus
Origin in Brain:	Medulla
Function:	Heart (sensory), Blood vessels (motor), Viscera (motor), Pharynx (motor), Larynx (sensory-motor).
Neurological Test:	See above mentioned technique for the determination of pharyngeal malfunction.

Number of Nerve:	XI.
Name of Nerve:	Spinal accessory
Origin in Brain:	Medulla
Function:	Neck muscles and Viscera (motor)
Neurological Test:	Check contours of head, neck and shoulders for normal appearance. Have client turn head against resistance, i.e., examiner places hand on each side of head and client tries to turn head against a moderate opposing pressure exerted by examiner. Normal if he can turn— suggestive of defect if he cannot or is very weak.

Number of Nerve:	XII.
Name of Nerve:	Hypoglossal
Origin in Brain:	Medulla
Function:	Tongue muscles (motor)
Neurological Test:	Have client protrude tongue—if it deviates, tongue will deviate to paralyzed side.

Chapter VI

CAUSES OF DYSFUNCTION

INTRODUCTION

T HERE ARE FOUR basic causes of non-verbalism in the young child: brain-injury, mental subnormality, emotional illness, and deafness.

Because of altered brain structure, the brain-injured child is often incapable of completely developing his communicative skills; for example, he may be only perceptually handicapped, or he may show signs of disturbed functioning in many areas. If language development is retarded, he is classified as an aphasic child.*

The mentally subnormal child cannot learn as much, or as rapidly, as his chronologically aged peers. His brain functioning is such that all abilities regarding the psychological events are depressed.

The emotionally ill child who manifests severe non-verbalism is essentially a psychotic child who, innately, may have well-

---

* There is apparently a good deal of confusion regarding the term aphasia and aphasoid when applied to the brain-injured child. The confusion seems to stem from the fact that some make a distinction between the child who has never spoken because of brain-damage and the child who has developed language but who has lost this capacity because of damage to the brain. The former is generally referred to as an aphasoid (aphasic-like) child while the latter condition is commonly called aphasia. It should be understood, however, that these terms mean different things to different people. It is the author's opinion that this is, however, a "distinction without a difference," and there is no reason why we cannot refer to these children as having "retarded language development because of congenital or acquired brain injury."

developed communicative abilities but doesn't "want" to use them.

The deaf child has a severe reduction of incoming sensory experiences and manifests communicative dysfunctions.

BRAIN INJURY

The syndrome presented by the minimally brain-injured child goes by a variety of names: cerebral dysfunction, encephalonic dysfunction, brain damage (as well as brain injury), etc. Recent literature emphasizes the nature of minimal brain injury as opposed to gross damage. It has been suggested by some writers that children who have been diagnosed as being emotionally ill, mentally retarded, or deaf are actually suffering from minimal brain-injury indicating a difficulty in differentially diagnosing these children.*

We do know, however, that the minimally brain-injured child may present impairment in one or more of the psychological events previously mentioned. The impairment may also affect only a facet of an event (e.g., only *visual* perception may be impaired).

If brain-injury is suspected because of the nature of the case-history, and/or tests, and/or observations, the child should be thoroughly examined. Not only may one or more of the psychological events be impaired but other functions may also show signs of impairment. For example, there may be present a behavioral disorder, and/or intellectual subnormality, and/or epilepsy. It is important for the therapist and parent to understand these problems if the child is to receive optimum help.

For this reason we now discuss these three problems:

A. *Epilepsy*—Epilepsy may be considered a "symptom" in

---

* In a speech presented to the Virginia Speech and Hearing Association in 1959, Dr. Jon Eisenson stated that many of his older colleagues feel that few non-verbal children are aphasic while many of his younger colleagues believe that they are. This statement and other written material indicate (see, for example, *The Concept of Congential Aphasia From The Standpoint of Dynamic Differential Diagnosis,* A Symposium, 34th Annual Convention, American Speech and Hearing Association, 1959) the difficulties involved in differentially diagnosing the cause of a child's non-verbalism.

which there are recurring lapses of unconsciousness, with or without convulsive manifestations, and varying greatly in frequency and severity. Convulsive disorders are often found in these children and may be of different types. Actually, more than a dozen seizure types have been identified and named according to symptoms. An epileptic seizure is produced by spontaneous local activity of nerve cells, beginning with a small area of gray matter and spreading to adjacent cells. This state of abnormal activity may remain localized and eventually "die out," or it may spread across the surface of the cortex. Pronounced brain wave alterations in the electro-encephalogram may be detected during the seizures.* There are three main types of seizures: grand-mal, petite-mal, and epileptic equivalent.

In a grand-mal seizure the patient may have a signal that an attack is impending. This warning may consist of a sensation of nausea, numbness, odor, unusual image, or flash of memory. For example, one adult patient revealed that immediately preceding each of his seizures, he had a "flash recollection" of the hospital where his brain-surgery was performed. The patient usually loses consciousness, falls to the floor, and emits a cry. Convulsions follow, and the patient lies stiff and rigid for as long as a minute or two while the muscles are in a state of mild contraction. A clonic phase occurs, in which rhythmic, convulsive body movements are apparent. Loss of control of the bowels and bladder is frequent, and injuries to the tongue from biting are common. A period of stupor and sleep, usually an hour to four hours, generally follows. The patient is often not his "normal self" if

---

* The E. E. G. gives a graphic representation of the electrical activity of different parts of the cortex. For example, the alpha rhythm is obtained from the frontal lobes, and for those ten years of age or older, we normally expect to find between eight and twelve cycles/sec occurring. If the frontal lobe is injured the alpha rhythm, or number of cycles/sec, should be abnormal. There are many individuals who present abnormal E. E. G.'s but manifest no sign of epilepsy; conversely, all epileptics show abnormal E. E. G.'s.

awake, and has little recollection of events during this period. Upon recovery from the attack, the patient may be aware that it has occurred.

The petite mal seizure may be merely a very short loss of consciousness. The patient may seem momentarily inattentive to what is going on. He pauses, and then continues without being aware that a seizure has occurred.

Epileptic equivalents (or Psychomotor epilepsy) is characterized by a state of "confusion." The patient has no memory as to what occurs during an attack.

Immediately after an attack the epileptic may manifest signs of perseveration in speech and behavior characterized by repetition of sounds and words and a pattern of speech closely resembling clonic stuttering.

Causes of epilepsy are usually divided into two groups, symptomatic and idiopathic. Symptomatic seizures are directly related to an obvious defect or abnormality of the brain such as birth injuries associated with difficult labor, head wounds, cerebral abscess, cerebral tumor, scars left by cerebral hemorrhage, or blood clots. There are other physical conditions which occasionally give rise to convulsions including diabetes, kidney disease, and strychnine poisioning but these seizures are not considered truly epileptic. Idiopathic epilepsy is the result of an unidentified injury (of unknown origin) and may be attributed to metabolic disturbances of the brain (which, in itself, may be familial or inherited).

If epilepsy is suspected, the therapist should be prepared for a seizure in the therapy room. If a grand-mal seizure occurs, the patient should be laid flat on the floor or couch with a folded coat or pillow under his head. Tight clothing should be lossened and the space around him cleared to prevent bruising of his limbs. No attempt should be made to restrain the convulsions unless he is hurting himself and it should then be done as gently as possible by grasping the victim's hands. The head can be tilted to one side, allowing the saliva or regurgitation to flow from the mouth. If the patient is seen at the beginning of the attack, a knotted handkerchief can be slipped between the teeth. A "cloth covered" tongue depressor can also be used. It is important that it be covered so that the patient cannot bite it, breaking it into splinters in the mouth. Once the seizure is over, the patient should rest until he wakes up "naturally." He should not be left unobserved until he is fully conscious, as he may remain in a confused or drowsy state. Nothing should be given by mouth until the patient is fully conscious.

Petite-mal attacks require no assistance.

B. *Behavioral Disorders*—The brain damaged child may manifest a behavioral disorder characterized by distractibility, disinhibition, hyperactivity, perseveration, and hyper-emotionality. *All young children manifest these conditions; they become abnormal when their degree of manifestation is "over and above" that which characterizes the "normal child."*

The brain injured child's "field" is primarily unstructured. This lack of structure has both the effect of increasing the relative intensity of extraneous stimuli and of also reducing the ability to attend to the desired stimulus. As previously stated, this may be due to his supersensitivity to stimuli and a concomitant difficulty in "tuning-out" to unwanted stimuli. This behavior is called distractibility and is often characteristic of the brain injured child.

The problem of disinhibition is closely related to distractibility. The child makes responses which are inadequate to the situation and which the normal child would not make because he would recognize their inadequacy. If a child, for example, is irritated by another child, he might throw an object at the other child. He may be able to explain why he should not have behaved in this manner, but in similar situations, he might repeat this behavior. It seems probable that we do not inhibit responses directly but that we avoid a particular response through selection of a more adequate one. This is the theory behind modern educational practices. We no longer say "Don't do this." or "Don't do that," but we try to provide the child with a choice reaction that will prove more adequate than the response which we wish to discourage. Before this substitution can be undertaken, the child must be aware of other possibilities and their consequences. This depends on his ability to structure both his perceptual and conceptual fields. The brain-injured child has particular difficulty when such relationships are involved since he is often impaired in his perceptual and conceptual abilities. This might account for his disinhibition.

Hyperactivity that is characterized by random, purposeless movement is often seen in the brain-injured child. Such behavior may be caused by the child's distractibility. It may also be related to a motor compulsiveness that cannot be controlled.

The brain-injured child has difficulty in changing rapidly from the evaluation of one set of relationships to another because he does not have the ability to restructure situations as rapidly as his normal peer. When a response is demanded, he responds on the basis of a structure he has developed previously. This is perseveration. This response has worked before, therefore, the child uses it with the hope that it will work again (thus perseveration differs from disinhibition because of the "success" factor). A child sometimes continues a line of behavior until he is interrupted or exhausted.

The brain damaged child is likely to "fly off the handle" without normal provocation. His emotionality is abnormal when he is faced with a situation which is too difficult and for which past experience furnishes him no basis for solution. He may laugh or cry catastrophically; he may go into a terrible "rage" or temper tantrum, etc. His

frustration tolerance is too low to allow him to cope with
the unexpected or difficult situations.

C. *Intellectual Sub-normality*—Damage to the brain could
well result in mental subnormality since the brain is the
seat of intelligence. A child so affected will probably
receive differential scores on the various sub-tests of an
intelligence test, suggesting that the damage has impaired specific, but not necessarily all, mental functions.
This problem will be more thoroughly discussed in the
next topic: Mental Subnormality.

MENTAL SUBNORMALITY

1. *Intelligence*—When we speak of intelligence, we refer to
the child's capabilities to learn (biological capacity), the
amount of learning that has taken place, and the use he
makes of this learning. All are determined, in varying
degrees, by psychometric tests.

Intelligence, therefore, may be defined as that combination
of qualities which an intelligence test measures. There
are, however, different intelligence tests that contain different content matter. It is quite possible, for example,
for a person to score above-average on one intelligence
test, average on another test, and below-average on a third
test. He may have scored highly on one test because it was
weighted with verbal tasks, and poorly on another test
because it was weighted with performance items. It is
always important, therefore, to know the nature and
content of the test used.

Some authorities have estimated that there are more than
100 different specific "intelligences." There is often or
usually a high correlation among the various intelligences;
that is, a certain score representing one intelligence may
well hold true for other untested intelligences, but this
need not necessarily be the case. In fact, it is usually not
the case when brain-injured children are tested.

2. *Causes of Mental Subnormality*—Mental subnormality is
caused by some alteration of structure or function of the

brain; the causes of these alterations, however, are more complex.

A. *Inheritance*

    1. Factors directly affecting the brain—We all inherit, through our parental genes,* a unique brain structure as well as function, that gives us our intellectual potential. Consequently, we have individual differences in innate intellectual ability. There are certain combinations of inherited genes that cause an aberrant brain structure and result in intellectual deficiencies. We believe, however, that a more common cause of "familial" retardation is the inheritance of sub-standard living conditions, poor prenatal care, and lack of opportunity. Such financial and environmental deprivation causes apathy that results in abnormal brain functioning. The President's Panel on Retardation reported that in approximately seventy-five to eighty-five per cent of the cases of retardation, etiological factors are unknown but that the vast majority of these cases come from the lower socio-economic bracket. (1) We believe, therefore, that many cases commonly referred to as "familial" or "garden variety," may well be a product of such deprivation. We do not believe that mental subnormality, per se, is inherited—contrary to the commonly quoted studies such as the Juke family or others—but rather an impaired brain structure or function; the former because of biological reasons and the latter due to social neglect.

    2. *Factors indirectly affecting the brain*—There are certain inheritable conditions (usually recessive traits) that cause some physiological alteration of

---

* The term "gene" is a convenient symbol; however, we know that the "stuff" that heredity is made of is chemical in nature and composed of D. N. A. and R. N. A. Once the chemical code is decoded and man is able to replicate the code, we shall be well on our way to creating life.

body functioning which, in turn, affects the brain. For example, Phenylketonuria (PKU) and Galactosemia are both conditions that affect protein metabolism; in the first case proper liver metabolism of phenylketonuria (an acid) is impaired and in the latter case, a carbohydrate, galactose, is improperly converted. These conditions are inherited. In both cases, brain functioning is affected and retardation results. There are probably other conditions, similar to these, in which there is improper functioning due to some inheritable trait; these conditions may be due to improper protein metabolism, or to abnormalities of the vascular system, e.g., the R.H. factor.

In 1940 Landsteiner and Wiener reported the presence of certain blood proteins that are incompatible and cause damage to the hemoglobin in the blood. Their work was performed on the Rhesus monkey and hence they called the proteins Rh+ (positive) and Rh— (negative). Approximately eighty-six per cent of the population contains the positive factor and fourteen per cent the negative factor. When an Rh— female bears a child conceived by an Rh+ male (and only this combination), there is danger that the incompatibility that results will destroy much of the hemoglobin in the blood and cause anoxia. (Oxygen unites with hemoglobin to form oxyhemoglobin, and in this state it is transmitted to the various cells of our body.) The first part of the body affected by anoxia is usually the brain. With each progressive pregnancy, the chance of more extreme damage becomes greater; there is usually no such problem with the first pregnancy unless the female has received a transfusion of Rh+ blood sometime in her past. This condition can be obviated by immediately transfusing the babies' blood.

B. *Chromosomal alterations**—The chromosomes (carriers of our genes) are forty-six in number; we each carry twenty-three from our mother and twenty-three from our father. These chromosomes "pair-up" in the conceptus according to their respective size, shape, etc.; there are, in the normal conceptus, twenty-three pairs of chromosomes. Recently, it has been found that there are, in some cases, extra chromosomes that attach themselves to the normal pairs and cause certain abnormalities in the offspring; for example, Mongolism (Down's Syndrome) is caused (most commonly) by an extra chromosome at the twenty-first pair. Similarly, Klinefelter's syndrome is caused by an abnormal number of sex chromosomes, resulting in feminine characteristics in the male, as well as mental retardation. Conversely, Turner's syndrome causes masculine characteristics to appear in the female, and is also accompanied by mental retardation. Although we do not know what causes the appearance of the extra chromosome, there is a higher incidence of Mongolism in mothers past the age of thirty-five. The female has a definite supply of eggs in her ovaries at birth and past a certain age (e.g., thirty-five) the eggs may become "old" and unstable. It has been suggested that some chromosomal problems are caused by "old eggs" in the female. Conversely, the male constantly regenerates new sperm. There are two other causes of mongolism, both rare, and both related to chromosome abnormalities; (1) translocation, where extra chromosome 21 material translocates and fuses with the 15th chromosome producing an abnormally large chromosome. This condition is familial and is the

---

* An interesting thesis is presented in Rachel Carson's *The Silent Spring,* relating some alterations of chromosomes to the frequent use of pesticides in our society.

only cause of mongolism that is inherited. (2) Mosaicism, where there are different chromosome counts in the different cells; that is, blood cells show a certain number of chromosomes while skin cells show a different number of chromosomes, etc.

C. *Brain Pathology*—Severe retardation often accompanies severe brain-injury; thus many custodial type retardates are severely brain-injured. The minimally brain injured child, on the other hand, is not really a retarded child as compared to other types of retardates. In minimal brain damage, one or more of the facets of intelligence is impaired but rarely is there an overall lowering of his potential. Furthermore, this type child is often habilitable to a normal or near-normal level.

The severity and extent of the brain-injury, therefore, is a significant prognostic factor. Severe injuries are often results of severe cases of anoxia, accidents that cause extensive damage to the brain, prolonged infectious disease affecting the brain (e.g., meningitis that goes untreated for any length of time). Minimal damage is often a result of mild cases of anoxia and so on. Similarly, thyroid atrophy, as found in cretinism, can cause varying degrees of mental subnormality.

Usually, an endogenous retardate (types A and B, aforementioned) will obtain similar scores on the various sub-tests of an intelligence test, and a statement of his I.Q. is meaningful because it indicates his overall potential and level of achievement. The exogenous retardate (type C) will usually receive differential scores on these sub-tests and a statement regarding his I.Q. is often meaningless (excluding cretinism).

A significant discrepancy among the various sub-tests or among performance and verbal scores is often suggestive of organicity, especially when the performance score is significantly lower than the verbal score.

3. Translation of the *Weschler Intelligence Scale for Children* Sub-Tests—One of the better intelligence tests than can be given to the retardate is the Weschler; this test allows for a clinical interpretation of the patient's problem. For this reason the following information is given:

1. *Verbal Scale*

   a. *Information*—memory of distant events; educational and cultural interests; general information; e.g., "How many weeks are there in a year?"

   b. *Comprehension*—judgment, social awareness, etc.; e.g., "Why are laws necessary?"

   c. *Digit Span*—immediate recall; e.g., digits are repeated forward and backwards; the examiner says 3-2-6, the patient is asked to repeat them as given and then backwards, i.e., 6-2-3.

   NORMS

Age	Number of Digits
3	3
4	4
7	5
10	6
14	7
18	8

   d. *Arithmetic*—ability to concentrate, mental alertness, etc.; e.g., "How much is $2 + 2$?", etc.

   e. *Similarities*—verbal concept formation, capacity for verbal abstraction; e.g., identification of "likeness" between different objects such as a dog and lion— why are they related?

   f. *Vocabulary*—educational level, best single test of general verbal intelligence (witness the number of paper and pencil vocabulary intelligence tests: #Peabody, Full Range, etc.).

2. *Performance Scale*

   a. *Picture arrangement*—ability to anticipate initial acts

or situations; e.g., a series of pictures are to be arranged to make for *logical* sequences.

b. *Block design*—tests visual motor coordination (eye-hand) and color discrimination; e.g., using colored blocks, the individual makes designs shown by the examiner.

c. *Picture completion*—ability to differentiate essential from non-essential; e.g., part of a picture is missing and the patient is to indicate the missing part.

d. *Object assembly*—test figure-ground ability, integrative abilities, visual (eye)—motor (hand); e.g., patient is given a number of flat cardboard pieces which he must fit together to make a face or any common object.

e. *Digit symbol*—capacity for new learning; e.g., the patient is shown some symbols associated with numerals; within a given time he must copy the symbols.

THE EMOTIONALLY ILL CHILD

Causes of emotional disorders are legion; in essence, however, we can categorize them into three main groups; (1) the immature child; (2) the neurotic child, and (3) the psychotic child. We are primarily concerned with the psychotic child.

The cause of psychosis in young children is vague. Many authorities, however, are coming to the conclusion that childhood schizophrenia and autism are caused by bio-chemicals that affect brain functioning and cause mal-adjustive personality characteristics. (There are many, however, who also believe that a "common denominator" found in all these children is a "cold" home environment; an environment where the parents are preoccupied and hence limited in their interaction with their child.)

Serotin, a bio-chemical has been found in the blood of adult schizophrenics and is thought to be intimately related to this form of psychosis since it is not found in the blood of non-schizophrenics. It is quite possible that metabolic disturbances or alterations that are genetically transmitted may cause an overproduction or under-production of certain chemicals that, in turn, affect brain functioning and affect personality development.

Although many people consider childhood schizophrenia and autism as distinct entities, for our purposes they may be considered as one and the same. Basically, both cause the child to be lacking in proper expressions of affective tone; the child does not laugh or cry or relate to his environment as would his normal peer. The child tends to be a "loner," he plays by himself and lives in a world of his own creation. His speech may be characterized by an echolalia (repetitions) and/or neologisms (coining of "new" words).

Often-times, "pre-psychotic behavior" is seen in these youngsters whereby they maintain some degree of contact with reality although their interactions are often bizarre.

A classic case we saw, sometime ago, was a youngster originally diagnosed as being severely mentally retarded. Our observation of her behavior led us to believe that she was schizophrenic. This child did not interact with her peer group and appeared to be in her "own world." By rewarding almost any behavior that she manifested, we have been able to partially draw her into "our world." To date this child has demonstrated a vocabulary of about 200 words; a result quite startling when one considers she had been a completely non-verbal child.

Personality development—By the term "emotional illness," we refer to mal-adjusted personalities. It is expedient for us, therefore, to discuss briefly some characteristics of personality development. The personality so unique to each individual emerges as a result of an interaction between his genetic endowment and his environment. From this interaction, we develop a self-concept or ego which becomes the reference point around which our experiences, attitudes, and adjustive reactions are organized.

The person who adjusts poorly to experiences, or who manifests asocial attitudes, is called a mal-adjusted person. An emotional disorder, characterized by any one or more of a variety of behavior disorders, is thus caused by poor or atypical adjustment to one's experiences.

Such adjustment patterns may be caused by abnormal genetic

endowment, environmental frustrations, or a combination of both factors. The former may relate to the inheritance of a "bad seed" per se, or more probably the inheritance of some factor which causes an alteration in the physiology or anatomy of the brain and, in turn, affects adjustive patterns. The latter is characterized by environmental frustrations and causes "needs" to go unfulfilled. A highly unpleasant state of anxiety is caused by these frustrations and in order to relieve oneself of these feelings, the individual often resorts to asocial adjustive patterns, the most primitive pattern being aggression.

THE DEAF CHILD

Deafness, or severe hearing loss, may be present either at birth or acquired post-natally. The most common etiology of a congenital nature is damage to the inner ear caused by hereditary nerve deafness; usually the cochlea is malformed or even absent. Since hereditary nerve deafness is a recessive trait, one in every four children of parents who carry the gene for deafness will be deaf. Equally common is congenital inner ear deficiency caused by measles and/or other diseases during the first trimester of pregnancy. Acquired or adventitious causes of deafness are also common, with disease toxemias heading the list. These and other causes of non-heredity deafness often result in multiple defects.

There are many other factors which may cause hearing problems but which do not affect the child in the same way as do the factors mentioned above.

Brain damage causing central deafness is one of these factors. This type of disorder is commonly characterized by the "aphasoid" condition reflected in an inconsistency of hearing; mental subnormality may be characterized by a general auditory disorder and may be due to congenital malformation of the auditory pathways; emotional disturbances may cause hysterical deafness. All of these kinds of hearing problems must be correctly diagnosed since appropriate treatment is dependent upon the proper diagnosis. None of these children, for example, belong in a school for the deaf. Yet, they are often found in such institutions simply because of incorrect diagnosis or, unfortunately, lack of any other agency to handle the problem.

Chapter VII

DIFFERENTIAL DIAGNOSIS

CASE-HISTORY DATA*

T HERE ARE FOUR basic areas of interest in case-history taking that are significant, relative to differential diagnosis: (1) the pregnancy; (2) birth; (3) immediate post-natal period, and (4) general post-natal development.

Many atypical events may take place during the pregnancy that may be significant (the student is referred to Ashley Montague's *Pre-Natal Influences,* a very readable source of information; see suggested readings). We are primarily concerned with three important areas: illnesses, general physical health, and the mother's emotional health. Research has shown that the probability of a mal-conceived child is greater when the mother has contracted any of a variety of infectious diseases during the first six months of pregnancy. We are concerned with the physical health of the mother in terms of her pre-natal care; that is, proper nutritional care, occupational hazards, exposure to undue radiation, etc. Poor emotional health as a causative factor is still controversial; however, there is apparently sufficient information to show cause for exploration of this area (see Strean, *The Normal Birth of Normal Babies,* as well as Montague's comments in *Pre-Natal Influences*). We are also concerned with parental ages at conception. Research, again, has shown that there is a higher incidence of abnormality when the mother is

------

* See Appendix 1 for sample forms used to collect case-history data.

past the optimum child-bearing age (middle twenties) or has not yet approached the optimum child-bearing age. Although most females' reproductive organs and systems are developed at puberty, they are not functionally operant (that is, they have difficulty conceiving) until they are approximately seventeen years of age. A pregnancy during those early years, however, is dangerous since the reproductive system is not yet completely capable of making the necessary changes to care for the conceptus. Consequently, we find a high incidence of abnormality in such offspring. This incidence gradually diminishes until we reach the optimum child-bearing years where it is at its lowest point. It gradually starts to rise again when the woman is past twenty-eight years of age and again shows a marked increase when she is past thirty-five years of age. There is no such comparable data concerning the male's age at conception; apparently the male age is not too important regarding its effects on the conceptus.

The embryonic insult most commonly and closely linked to brain-injury is pre-natal anoxia. It is known that oxygen is essential for the maintenance of life. The brain is most sensitive to lack of oxygen, and therefore, is most likely to be damaged when anoxia is present.

Anoxia may occur for four reasons. First, there may be mechanical factors preventing oxygen in the mother's blood from reaching the child. Examples of this are premature separation of the placenta, a twisted cord, or compression of the cord between the child and the mother's pelvis. Secondly, there may not be enough oxygen available. Severe anemia or a serious heart condition in the mother, hemorrhage during a threatened abortion, or premature separation of the placenta (up to the fourth month of pregnancy) may limit the oxygen supply for the infant. A third cause of anoxia is decreased maternal blood pressure. Serious and lengthy hypertension in the mother or Rh incompatability may result in the inability of the blood stream to carry sufficient oxygen. Last, toxins may make it impossible for the brain cells to use available oxygen.

In eliciting information about the birth of the child, we ask the following:

1. Term of pregnancy—normal term is nine months plus or minus two weeks. Research has shown that pre-mature babies (twins are often premature), especially those premature by more than a month, are born with a higher incidence of brain-injury caused by anoxia and/or hemorrhage. The cerebral vessels of the premature infant are fragile and the sudden change in pressure during birth may cause hemorrhaging. Similarly, post-term babies (those significantly delayed) show a higher incidence of brain-injury which may be due to their overly-large size and the consequent difficulties during the presentation of the head through the birth canal.

2. Twelve to eighteen hours of labor is normal for the first born, whereas the normal period of labor for succeeding births is eight to twelve hours. A precipitous or overly-long labor period may have significant ramifications in terms of the child's development. It is, however, difficult to obtain a true estimate of the labor period from the mother and care should be taken that the mother understands that you are concerned with the *first* indication of labor (and not when rhythmical and consistent labor pains were initiated).

3. Normal birth weight is between five to nine pounds, the average being around seven pounds. A baby is considered to be premature if his birth weight is less than five pounds and post-mature if more than nine pounds. Research indicates that the amount of neurological damage increases as the birth weight of the baby decreases (below five pounds), while a baby weighing more than nine pounds also often suffers from neurological damage due to prolonged labor often associated with above-average birth weight.

4. Normal presentation of the child is initiated, of course, by the emergence of the head; when the buttocks or feet come first, this is called a breech birth. When the normal birth process is not medically advisable, a caesarean section is performed. Any deviation from the normal

birth process should be questioned. The probability of damage is higher in abnormal deliveries.

5. The interviewer should be concerned with the possibility of a dry birth. If the amniotic sac breaks *any significant amount of time* before the child is born, there is a greater possibility of damage due to physical abuse and possible nutritional deprivation (the amniotic fluid not only acts as a "cushion" for the conceptus but also supplies nutrients and absorbs eliminative waste products).

6. If the umbilical cord is so arranged that it is gathered around the baby's neck, it may cause strangulation and hence anoxia.

7. Delayed breathing is pertinent. Although there is no need to hurriedly cut the umbilical cord (while attached, the baby still has his physical needs supplied), once cut, the baby must initiate respiration using his respiratory mechanism. At times, breathing is delayed for a variety of reasons, and if this delay is overly long it can cause anoxia.

An informal study performed at our Speech and Hearing Clinic involved the compilation of significant data (from our inactive case-histories) pertinent to this discussion. Unfortunately, we were unable to relate these data to the type of abnormality.

The following was revealed:

Mother's Age at Birth of Child	No.	Father's Age at Birth of Child	No.	Type of Birth	No.	Patients' Sex	No.	Weight	No.
14	1	17	2	Normal	431	Male	460	2	1
15	0	18	2	Breech	16	Female	192	2½	2
16	0	19	4	Cesarean	17			3	3
17	5	20	3	Other	30			3½	5
18	15	21	5					4	14
19	18	22	17					4½	3
20	29	23	18					5	3
21	24	24	31					5½	14
22	31	25	42					6	33
23	27	26	29					6½	24
24	34	27	32					7	82
25	39	28	37					7½	50
26	33	29	31					8	36
27	20	30	16					8½	19
28	19	31	34					9	9
29	16	32	20					9½	7
30	18	33	8					10	2
31	23	34	29					10½	1
32	15	35	14					11	1
33	17	36	21					11½	0
34	10	37	16					12	0
35	12	38	14					Over 12	1
36	6	39	17						
37	9	40	13						
38	6	41	8						
39	3	42	10						
40	9	43	3						
41	1	44	6						
42	4	45	2						
43	2	46	1						
44	1	47	0						
45	0	48	1						
46	1	49	1						
47	0	50	0						
48	0	Above 50	17						
49	0								
50	1								
Above 50	0								

The immediate post-natal history can often reveal pertinent information:

1. Ask if the mother noticed any scars, bruises, or deformities when she first saw the child. Occasionally, an instrumental delivery causes physical damage to the head (although this is rarer than was once believed).
2. One should probe into the possibility of seizures or convulsions. Most parents recognize the grand-mal type seizure, but they often tend to miss the lesser forms of convulsive attacks.
3. Feeding difficulties should be explored. Although the most likely cause of a feeding problem is an incompatible formula, the possibility of a paresis or paralysis of the mechanism involved in deglutition should not be ignored. Such a condition may be symptomatic of a larger syndrome caused by brain-injury.
4 The normal hue of the new-born is reddish-pink. Occasionally a yellowish tinge is found in the new-born suggestive of jaundice. While this condition is normal in the neonate, it becomes abnormal if it appears some months after birth. The most common abnormality of skin coloring is caused by the frequently mentioned anoxia which causes a bluish color.

When obtaining information about the general development of the child, there are a number of areas that should be explored:

1. Maturational development should be investigated. Data should be obtained concerning the ages when the child was able to perform certain tasks such as walking, talking, etc. (for detailed information relative to these norms, the student is referred to Gessel and Ilg, *The Child's First Five Years* and/or their companion book, *The Child From Five To Ten* which also summarizes the first five years; also see the developmental history form in the appendix). Any significant delay in this area should be noted and thoroughly explored since there is an inextricable interrelationship between maturational level and neurological functioning.

Such delays are often symptomatic of brain-injury and/or mental subnormality (and sometimes emotional illness). To comprehensively test the child's social maturity, the Vineland Social Maturity Scale should be used. This test, in part, is based on maturational development.

2. The child's illnesses are important only if they reveal a change in his behavior after his illness as compared to premorbid behavior. Fevers with high temperatures (past 105°) are frequent causes of minimal brain-injury and should be regarded with suspicion.

3. The auditory behavior of the child should be explored. Inconsistencies in hearing are often found in youngsters who have normal hearing abilities but who are passing through a negativistic stage and just don't want to respond. Oftentimes, they appear to be deaf or hard-of-hearing. We are concerned, however, with the child who is truly inconsistent in his hearing; a detailed investigation will often reveal if the inconsistency is a real problem. If an examination proves the latter, it is suggestive of brain-injury causing auditory imperception (or auditory agnosia and/or auditory aphasia). Inquire from the parents when the child first babbled, and investigate whether or not his babbling became inflected and then socialized (vocal play). Absence of inflection and socialization might indicate deafness, since the deaf child, not hearing himself, does not pass through these stages. The parent should be asked if the child seems to look at a sound source, e.g., the mother upon speaking to the child, or an unexpected (or deliberate) loud noise in his environment.

4. The child's behavior is another area to be investigated. The psychotic child shows disturbances of affective-tone or emotionality; he may cry or laugh excessively and without apparent cause, or conversely, he may not show any emotionality; he tends to withdraw and prefers to be by himself. These children are often thought to be retarded because of their withdrawal type behavior, but

careful observation by the parent reveals abilities that the retarded do not (or should not) develop at their chronological age. The brain-injured often present a syndrome of mal-behavior that is most difficult for parents to cope with, such as hyperactivity and distractibility; one should be sure that this aberrant behavior is not confused with the normal child's manifestation of this twin behavioral problem (all children are hyperactive and distractible to some degree). By asking parents to compare their child's behavior with that of a sibling or friend of an approximate chronological age, one can often obtain reliable information. There are other forms of mal-behavior sometimes seen in the brain-injured child that are discussed elsewhere in this book.

TESTS

Numerous formal and informal tests can be given to the patient, most of which have been previously mentioned.

OBSERVATION OF BEHAVIOR

Perhaps the most important technique at our disposal allowing for proper diagnosis is observation of behavior. The experienced therapist rules-out improbable etiologies upon observing specific types of behavior.

The following chart serves to summarize the behavioral anomalies:

	Brain-damage	Mental Subnormality	Emotional Illness E.G., Autism	The Deaf
Verbal Language (receptive and/or expressive)	May be retarded (if so, called an aphasia)	Retarded	Retarded	Retarded
Vocalization 1. Quality	good	good	good	distorted quality
2. Vocal play and/or Jargon and/or Echolalia	normal development	delayed development	normal development	absent
Gestures	normal	may be used	may be used for fantasy but not for communication	used extensively
Response to Sound	may or may not be inconsistent	responds consistently to concrete but may ignore abstract sounds	responds in indirect manner	consistent when threshold is reached
Sensitivity to Visual and Tactile Clues	may be reduced or may be very sensitive	may be reduced	rejects	very sensitive to both
Motor Behavior	hyperactive, distractible, perseveration, catastrophic responses	normal; if atypical behavior is found may be due to frustrations and will be different, in kind, from brain-injured (which are random and pointless)	may be stereotyped	may be excessive body movement to keep in contact with visual clues
Motor Development	may or may not be retarded	retarded	normal	normal
Social Maturity (use Vineland Social Maturity Scale)	may be severely or slightly retarded	immature-consistent with mental abilities	deficient-ignores others	limited to visually perceived situations

	Brain-damage	Mental Subnormality	Emotional Illness E.G., Autism	The Deaf
Emotional Behavior	may be quite mal-adjusted	asocial behavior due to frustrations	usual withdrawal but may display aggressiveness or catastrophic behavior at times	often immature reaction to frustrations
Formal Intelligence Tests	1) gap between verbal and performance; performance being lower 2) more inconsistent on the various sub-tests due to mal-function of one or more of the various stages in development	general retardation in both verbal and performance tests; similar scores on all sub-tests	may have better performance score than verbal score	some retardation; especially on those tasks related to hearing. Special tests are required

In summary, our first concern is the determination of significant retardation in language development. This is done by one or more of the language tests we have discussed. Our next concern is the determination of the cause of the non-verbalism. This is done by using case-history data, test information, and observation of behavior. Always keep in mind the four possible causes of non-verbalism and continually try to rule-out these possibilities on the basis of the information you have been able to gather.

Chapter VIII

HABILITATION

INTRODUCTION

It is our philosophy that the non-verbal child, who also presents a syndrome of disordered functioning, is best treated in a center where he can receive his education and those therapies that are beneficial to his habilitation; a program that is intensive and multi-disciplined; a program whereby all of the child's needs are fulfilled. To this end, we envision a center that maintains a nursery and kindergarten program, a school program, vocational education, and varied therapeutic programs. The child is enrolled in this "total" program when quite young (two and one-half years of age if possible) and continues in it until he is capable of becoming a relatively independent member of his community.

SOME GENERAL INFORMATION

Before we can professionally treat a child's needs, we must be aware of what his needs are. This can only be accomplished after a correct diagnosis has been obtained. Even then, however, a child cannot be helped to achieve his potential until any stumbling blocks which might impede progress are removed from our therapeutic path. Behavior problems, for example, and especially those often seen in the brain-injured child, must first be obviated if learning is to take place. The child cannot *retain* stimuli if he cannot *attend* to the stimuli (or experience) for a sufficient length of time. Similarly, the deaf child must be given improved channels (and/or "new" channels should be developed) through which he can learn.

No rigid habilitation program can be devised for any group of children; rather each child must have an individual program that is "geared" to his individual needs. We do not mean to imply that each child will need all of the therapies discussed in the following pages. We are of the opinion, however, that many of these children exhibit different kinds of minimal problems. These problems, because of their minimal nature, often go undiagnosed and untreated. Their lack of treatment handicaps the therapist and impedes progress. We are suggesting, therefore, that it may be beneficial if doubtful cases, or those cases in which a "weakness" is evidenced in "other" communicative skills, received therapy in these skills.

Intensive parental counseling is an important adjunct to a successful program. Many parents have a tendency to over-protect their handicapped children. Removing such a parental handicap is a pre-requisite for effective therapy. Many of these children have untapped potential that will never be fully developed unless the parents cooperate in this endeavor.

For more effective treatment, it is desirable to have a physical plant designed to cater to the individual problems of the patients (2, 13).

Children with behavior problems due to brain-injury are best treated in rooms that eliminate extraneous stimuli. This can be accomplished by temporarily converting a sound-proof room (or any room that is relatively free from sound) into a therapy room. At the same time use only one light bulb to illuminate the room. In such a manner, extraneous auditory and visual stimuli can be kept to a minimum.

The therapist should wear simple clothing that would not be too distracting; furthermore, any distracting jewelry should be removed from the body before initiating therapy.

Initially, the child should receive individual therapy in this type environment; gradually, the therapist might expose the child (under controlled conditions) to some distracting stimuli. When the child can tolerate them without manifesting distractibility, or any form of deviant behavior, he might then be ready for a group situation.

This treatment varies from that of the retardate who needs many visual-aids in his environment. However, any child who is hyperactive and distractible can best be treated in the manner suggested above.

The autistic child can best be treated in a room where the therapist can afford to be permissive; where fairly rigid rules regarding behavior, often necessary for the brain-injured or retardate, are not required. In essence, a specially designed play therapy room is desirable. Here the therapist can liberally reward behavior, almost any kind of behavior, in an attempt to get the child to socialize.

The deaf child (pre-school) needs auditory training equipment as well as numerous visual aids. His room design need not be significantly different from any other child's except that he needs good lighting for lip-reading purposes.

SPECIFIC THERAPEUTIC TECHNIQUES

Hearing-Auditory Training

Auditory training is the process of teaching the hard-of-hearing child or adult to take full advantage of the sound clues which are still available to him. It is aimed at improving communication through the systematic use of residual hearing potential. The child who is trained to use his residual hearing to the fullest extent develops a better understanding of the relationships between sounds and objects, sounds and actions, and sounds and people. When hearing is faulty, development of speech is likely to be retarded or imperfect. The child learns faulty interpretations of sound or he learns to substitute other senses for the ear. Vision and touch tend to become his primary means of receiving communication. Gestures tend to replace speech as the method of communicating with other people. Therefore, if there is any suspicion that a baby is hard-of hearing, his early years must be filled with loud and varied sounds. Auditory training assumes the extremely important role of making the child appreciate sound and want to hear it.

The listening act is made up of at least two functions: the first is the conveyance of an auditory signal to the sensory receiving station in the brain, and the second is the recognition and inter-pretation of that signal. Physiological hearing alone, even when highly trained and aided by an amplifying device, does not provide a magic key to understanding. It must be fortified by the help of sight, touch and muscle sensation. Nor is listening a matter of recognition of sound alone. Such factors as intensity, rhythm, inflection and mood all change the meaning of simple sounds. It becomes necessary, then, to awaken in the child an awareness of these things.

Techniques in auditory training are designed not only to stimulate response to sound, but to improve the child's whole response to his environment. Auditory training, over a period of time, enables the parent and the teacher to estimate more accurately the nature and degree of the hearing loss and its relation to the child's future education. To expect a standard set of responses from all deaf children provides only a false basis on which to make a diagnosis.

It is important to remember that auditory training may be a long and slow process. The very young child has no conception of what "listening" means and it becomes necessary to give him a pleasant and enjoyable first experience of it. In the case of the very young deaf child, the unaided voice should be used at first. The young child who cannot understand the reason for wearing earphones may permit the parent or the teacher to talk near his ear in a normal tone of voice. Many deaf children will accept the wearing of earphones within a short period of time, but there are those who need more time, sometimes months, and both parent and therapist must be prepared for this possibility and be willing to give the child time to adjust to the use of earphones and to amplified sound. If the child rejects all auditory training consist-ently, even violently, the therapist should compare this attitude with the child's reactions to other phases of the training, and should try to determine whether the rejection is for auditory training only, or involves other factors such as parent-child relationships.

Occasionally a child who has some usable hearing will react in an exaggerated way to amplified sound. The parent and the

therapist have to take precautions with this child. He has difficulty in adjusting to the sounds he hears, and during the early
weeks of training he is not able to tolerate much amplification.
If he will use the headset, he should be watched carefully for
signs of nervousness and fatigue. Therapy sessions should
be short, and very gradually increased. Auditory training
should be offered whenever the child will accept it, not only
during formal lesson periods. Parents have found that they get
good results when lying beside the child on the bed before he
goes to sleep at night, when he is at ease, and when his whole
body is touching that of the speaker so that he is more aware of
vibrations. Auditory training is more effective when it is combined with lip-reading, speech preparation and other activities.

The *objectives* of *auditory training* that are potentially attain-
able for deaf children (losses above 80 or 90 db) are:

1. *Improvement in speech perception.* These children are
   not likely to achieve any appreciable level of auditory
   discrimination for speech, at least to the point where they
   can understand connected language through hearing
   alone. However, they can be taught to appreciate the
   temporal patterns of speech and to improve control of
   the intensity, and in some instances of the pitch, of the
   voice. Speech perception is improved through auditory
   training, particularly when it is combined with lip-reading.
   Failure to make improvement in communication through
   speech may be attributed to the fact that the training was
   not begun early enough, actually in the first year of life.
2. *Improvement in emotional behavior.* Many frustrations
   are encountered by the deaf or severely hard-of-hearing
   child because of his inability to interact well with his
   hearing peers. Auditory training often attenuates this
   problem.

The four major steps of auditory training for deaf children
are: (1) the development of awareness of sound; (2) the
development of gross discrimination; (3) the development of
broad discrimination among simple speech patterns, and (4) the
development of finer discrimination of speech. It is important to

realize that the child must form the "habit of listening." Even the very young child under two should be talked and sung to close to his ear, and he should be encouraged to look at and to listen to sound-producing objects. This is the first stage of auditory training. As the child matures, he needs to develop an awareness for the sound and the realization that it can have meaning. It is essential that the child be surrounded by sounds that are intense enough to be sensed.

All lessons in auditory training for the deaf child have a common goal—the better understanding of speech. Each lesson has a specific aim, with the beginning lessons concentrating on awareness of sound. The child must be taught to direct his attention to sounds, learning that they are meaningful and often enjoyable. This can best be accomplished by presenting those sounds which he can relate to his own experience. An approach through play is particularly useful because it builds on enjoyment, without disapproval and punishment, and is very helpful in penetrating his resistance to listening. The child should be surrounded with loud sounds that are related to his everyday activities.

The therapist should then initiate a plan whereby the child is taught to recognize and discriminate among gross sounds (non-speech sounds). Such discrimination can be developed by using sound-producing objects representative of these stimuli (e.g., toy animals, etc.). The child first associates the object with the sound and is then called upon to indicate which object, activated out of his sight, produced the sound. Once the child has learned to identify highly dissimilar sounds by ear, sounds increasingly alike are used to refine the child's skills of discrimination. *One point needs to be particularly stressed.* The therapist must remember that the child is deaf and *not* hard-of-hearing; that although similar procedures are used for both types of children, they must be "tailor-made" to fit the needs of the deaf child. It should also be remembered that gross discriminations depend upon differences in frequency, in intensity, in sound composition, and in the sequences and patterns of these three acoustic elements. The training program must be planned to stress each of these factors, both independently and in various combinations.

The development of broad discriminations among simple speech patterns, the third step in auditory training, is a similar application of the techniques used to develop gross discriminations. Once the child has learned that sounds differ from one another, he is ready to start learning to understand speech. Again, training must start by teaching him to make distinctions that are easy (e.g., stressing differences in vowels). Another approach is to start the training in speech discrimination with a few meaningful phrases. Here the goal is to have the child recognize the whole phrase and assign meaning to it without analyzing its parts. Each phrase must be closely related to his everyday experiences. The advantage of this method is that it reproduces the normal manner of learning. As the phrases become more familiar, the words begin to emerge and assume meaning. Here the child is likely to develop an appreciation for auditory training because it is related to speech reception and expression.

Auditory training is not complete until the child has learned to make distinctions as exact as his hearing loss allows. Thus, the final stage of auditory training aims toward building increasingly precise discriminations, particularly for speech. The methods used depend partly on the child's general maturity and partly on his past accomplishments in learning to hear effectively. Basically, however, three kinds of skill must be taught.

First, encourage him to recognize the more subtle phonetic differences. Secondly, the child must be taught to know and understand a large vocabulary of spoken words. There must be both variety in the words and phrases used for practice and opportunity to fix the meaning of words through diverse experiences. Finally, the child needs training in understanding connected speech; that is, he must learn to integrate his growing vocabulary so that he understands phrases and sentences quickly and accurately. Even if the child never reaches the stage where he can make difficult speech discriminations, he should deliberately and continually be encouraged to listen to speech. Normal patterns of speech will furnish a guide for the rhythm and intonation of the child's own speech, which in the case of very deaf children needs every possible help to make it intelligible. It should be recognized that even at best, the deaf child will never attain *refined* speech patterns; rather, the goal should be the attainment of *intelligible* speech patterns.

For hard-of-hearing children, the potential for auditory training is greater than for deaf children. We may look for better development of gross discriminations of speech patterns and of speech sounds. Lip-reading is likely to be the supplementary (to hearing) means of communication for most hard-of-hearing children.

Persons whose hearing loss is great enough to cause disturbance in communication will likely wear, or be preparing to wear, a hearing aid. To this extent most work in auditory training will be related to the hearing aid. In preliminary training it is usually better to work with a non-wearable hearing aid to avoid the limitation of fidelity imposed by the size of wearable models. The child who responds well to auditory training, and whose voice and speech show improvement after auditory training with an amplifier, should be considered a candidate for a wearable aid. Any child who will accept such an aid, and who obviously could benefit from one, should have the opportunity of using it through as much of the day as is possible for him.

First lessons in hearing aid wearing should be happy occasions. Easy, familiar sounds, games and activities which make a child feel secure and successful in a new learning situation should be selected for this purpose. Several toys whose sound-producing mechanism can be seen and heard are used in different ways to stimulate a child's awareness of and interest in everyday sounds of his environment. Toys, producing sounds that differ in loudness, tone, and rhythm, offer an easy lesson in awareness and discrimination of sound. Each sound, reinforced by visible evidence of its production, can be identified successfully by most hearing aid wearers who are learning to look and listen.

In relation to the hearing aid, auditory training should promote negative adaptation to unwanted sound. Negative adaptation (or "tuning-out") is a matter of rejection of unwanted stimuli (noise). The best means of promoting this rejection should be a structured situation that demands a choice between wanted and unwanted sounds. This choice suggests an active listening rather than a passive listening activity. An active listening activity involves a response which allows a check on the accuracy of the listening. A passive listening practice would involve no such check or response.

Talker-listener drill or intelligibility testing, as a structure for auditory training for the hard-of-hearing, is advantageous for several reasons. All agencies that have studied speech intelligibility have concluded that taking a test improves both talking and listening ability. The test structure as a training scheme also affords motivation by making communication a game. It compels the listener to pay "close" attention to the sound stimuli if he is to receive a "good" score.

As has been previously stated, auditory training is of great value to the child who is hard-of-hearing or deaf. The following points should be kept in mind by the therapist:

1. Auditory training tends to be more effective when reinforced through other sensory systems.
2. The teaching techniques should be geared to a child's auditory potential.
3. Auditory training, with or without a hearing aid, should be initiated as soon as is possible.
4. Acceptance of hearing aids may be developed through differential auditory experiences that are meaningful; through the development of gross discrimination of various environmental sounds; and within the limits of the child's hearing, through the development of speech discrimination abilities.
5. The child should have the benefit of amplified sound in all of his classroom work, at home, and at play (whenever possible).
6. Children should be taught as early as possible the management and care of their hearing aids.

Perceptual Training

The child may be deficient in any one or more of his perceptual abilities; furthermore, the impairment may range in degree from mild to severe. The therapist must ascertain the area and the degree of involvement before initiating therapy. Some suggested therapies are as follows:

1. *Visual Perception*
    a. *Space*—develop a left to right sequence (a pre-reading skill) by the following:
        1. Arrange story pictures in a left to right sequence (may use flannel board).
        2. Arrange blocks or squares of colored paper of varying sizes, small to large, in a left to right sequence.
        3. Use peg and form board placing objects from left to right.
    b. *Figure-Ground*—the therapist's goal is to increase the patient's tolerance for distracting backgrounds (grey color seems to be least distracting), thereby increasing his awareness of the foreground. This might be accomplished in two ways: increase the "strength" of the background by using first, light lines, dots, and small figures, and then heavier lines, etc.; and second, gradually decrease the "strength" of the foreground by decreasing its size and using lighter shades of color.
    c. *Distance*—therapy can initially involve coloring or water painting. The objects to be painted can be drawn forms (circle, cross, triangle, square). If it was observed, during the testing session, that the child had difficulty in performing this task, the present need is to gradually get the child to color along the lines of the drawing. Practice in throwing balls at targets may also help develop better visual distance perception by developing accuracy and overcoming tendencies to overshoot or undershoot the targets. Another problem which may be found is an inability to recognize "near" and "far." Drills on observing which object is farthest away and which object is closest should be initiated. Gradually, the distance between the objects should be decreased until there is little difference. Both objects should be close, but one just a little farther away than the other.

d. *Color, Size, and Shape Perception*—the child should first learn to distinguish the primitive aspects of perception; i.e., color, size and shape. The therapist should have duplicates of different colors, sizes and shapes and encourage the child to match-discriminate among the stimuli. (An effective therapeutic "tool" is a color-form board, the pieces on one side being all the same color, the other side having different colored pieces matching specific grooves. These color-form pieces can also be made of different sizes enabling the therapist to work on color, size, and shape with one therapeutic aid.)

   1. *Shape*—many times it may be necessary and beneficial to help the child trace different geometric forms in order to obtain an awareness of the movement involved in making the forms. The therapy should continue until the child, when requested, selects the figure suggested by the therapist from the total grouping of all the many geometric forms.

   2. *Size*—this work should be done by having the child match the forms by size (small with small, large with large, etc.) until he can do it readily. A more advanced task would be to have the child match in sequential order such as small, large, larger, and so on.

   3. *Color*—therapy for the recognition of color should first involve the matching of different colored swatches of felt material or different colored pieces of cardboard. Only the primary colors should be used at first. As therapy progresses and success is experienced, additional colors should be added. Eventually, work may be introduced concerning the grouping of all shades of one color. Associating colors with objects may aid in recognition and retention of colors. For example, "See! It is *red* like my lipstick!" or "Can you show me something in the room that is green?"

e. *Form Perception*
   1. *Objects and Pictures*—Working with a doll house

and doll furniture may greatly benefit the child in recognizing the objects found in the home. A playhouse
which is divided into rooms provides possibilities for
good training and can be enjoyable at the same time.
Work can also involve having the child look for
objects which have been hidden in the room in order
to work on recognition and discrimination of objects.

2. *Letters and Numbers*—cards containing the letters of
   the alphabet (capital and lower case letters) should
   be used. There should be two sets of cards for
   capital letters and two sets of cards for lower case
   letters. One set should be printed, the other set
   should be written. Work with the letter cards should
   stress ready recognition through matching of the
   letters in all forms. A short retention span can also
   be increased by having the child point to, match, or
   pick up more than one card at a time. Similarly,
   number perception can be enhanced.

3. *Words*—therapy should consist of the matching of
   like words (printed) at first. Treatment should be
   aimed at progressing to the more abstract levels of
   matching words that mean the same, look the same,
   or sound the same. The written form of the word
   should gradually be added. Matching the word with
   its corresponding object is also desirable.

f. *Body-image*—the techniques, discussed in our testing
   section, can be used to evaluate the child's knowledge
   of his own body and how to control its parts. Impairment in any one or more of these abilities indicates the
   need for therapy. The type of therapy required is
   indicated by his abilities or lack of abilities in each test.

2. *Auditory Perception**

a. *Gross Sounds*—an inefficiency in this area indicates a
   need for drill in discriminating between types of sounds.
   Therapeutic techniques for improving discrimination

---

* See previous section on auditory training for more detailed information.

among environmental, animal, and musical sounds should be employed. Sound objects should be utilized until the child can recognize them in isolation. The therapist should then stress techniques to aid in selecting the appropriate sound-producing object from among several. The therapist should place several objects on a table in front of the child. With the child's eyes covered (or closed), the therapist produces a sound from one of the objects. The child should be instructed to open his eyes and identify the appropriate object. Eventually, therapy should progress to more abstract sources.

b. *Speech Sounds*—initially drill on recognition of and discrimination between the vowel and consonant sounds, then proceed to the discrimination of various consonant sounds, as indicated by the child's impairment. Have the child indicate whether the sounds are the same or different. Work should then progress gradually to the recognition and discrimination of words.

c. *Psychological Aspects of Sound*—the emphasis here is on discrimination between sounds of different pitches, different loudnesses, and different qualities. Have the patient indicate whether the stimuli are the same or different.

3. *Tactile Perception*

In this area, drill should be concentrated on the development of recognition and discrimination of objects by touch. The same procedures as those involved in testing should be used.

4. *Retention*

a. *Auditory*

1. Present numbers to the patient and ask him to repeat them; e.g., 2-4, 2-7-9, etc. Gradually increase sequences (either two or three or more numbers per presentation according to table of norms on page 39).
2. Present letters.
3. Present numbers and letters.

4. Present arithmetic problems, e.g., $2 + 2 - 1 = ?$.

5. Spell word; have patient say the word. Stay within certain categories, i.e., parts of the body.

b. *Visual*

1. By gesture (without auditory stimulation) instruct patient to point to the.....and the.....and the..... Gradually increase the number of stimuli.

Perceptual Motor Training

1. *Visual-motor*

   a. *Eye-hand*—show the child different colored geometric forms, letters, numbers and have him *trace* them in a sandbox, on a chalkboard, on paper, on sandpaper "cut-outs;" then have him *copy* them, and then *draw* them without copying; (2) throw rings on a stake, throw beanbags at holes in a board, etc.

   b. *Eye-leg*—hopping, skipping, jumping, walking rail, etc.

2. *Kinesthetic-motor*

   Develop kinesthetic awareness by having the child use affected muscle(s) without the benefit of the visual sense; for example, if tongue movements are awkward, have the child touch a tongue depressor placed in different positions around the lips without seeing the movement involved. If he has difficulty in performing this activity, let him watch himself in the mirror for visual guidance. Once this ability has been mastered, attempt the movement without the mirror. The same technique can be used by applying small dabs of peanut butter or small pieces of cornflakes in different parts of the mouth. The patient is asked to remove the peanut butter with his tongue and without visual guidance.

3. *Restricted Perceptual-motor Abilities*

   A number of children with impaired perceptual-motor abilities have restricted approaches to activities. They can be helped by exercises designed to foster different solutions to motor problems; e.g., going across a mat in different ways; i.e., crawling, walking, hopping, etc.

Concept-formation Training

Conceptual abilities can be enhanced by presenting dissimilar objects or pictures and asking the child to categorize them; e.g., the therapist might collect a number of pictures from various magazines typifying eating utensils, animals, musical instruments, parts of the body and so on. The therapist might then present four pictures, three of which are of eating utensils and ask the child to give him that picture which is different—the one that "doesn't belong" (and, if possible, have patient indicate *why* it doesn't belong here).

Similarly, a doll house can be used. Give the child both appropriate and inappropriate objects for placement. Can the child select and properly place those objects that belong in the house?

Parents can enhance this ability in their everyday interaction with the child by pointing out similarities between or among stimuli that constantly bombard the child, e.g.:

1. house—umbrella—they both keep you dry.
2. cat—truck—they both make sounds.
3. grass—tree—they both grow in the ground.
4. etc.

Language Training

There are two equally important philosophies pertinent to language habilitation. The Myklebust (Northwestern) technique and the McGinnis (CID) technique.

The Myklebust theory embraces three levels of language development; inner language in which the ability to understand and make proper use of environmental stimuli is developed, receptive language which allows one to understand symbols, and expressive language which enables one to use symbols.

The McGinnis technique stresses the perception and retention of phonemes that make up our language symbols. When a child can recognize and discriminate from among a number of phonemes, he is taught word concepts employing these phonemes. Monsees (9), who used the McGinnis method, writes as follows:

We start with the sound elements instead of words and phrases. The child is taught to recognize the letter symbols and to read the sounds the letters stand for. Then two or three sounds are put together to form a word. The word is written in two colors by the teacher, after a structured drill leading up to the word. The child reads the sounds in sequence from memory. Then the word is associated with a picture of the object it represents. The child traces the word on the blackboard—or copies it if he is able. The child then watches the teacher's lips as she says the word broken up and then smoothed directly into his ear or behind him if he is using a hearing aid; the child repeats the word, finds the picture, matches it to the written form and reads it aloud. Finally the child recalls the word from the picture alone and later writes the word from memory. All sensory channels are stressed for the purpose of achieving memory of the sounds that go into a word and these sounds in proper sequence; there is the visual reinforcement of the word written in colors with a change of color signaling a change of sound; visual kinesthetic through the experiences of tracing, copying, and writing the words; auditory through the presentation of the word through this channel of isolation. After a substantial number of nouns have been learned, the building of sentences and more complex language begins. When sufficient language has been mastered by the child, the lessons are based upon the regular academic school subjects to provide a well-rounded education program and to prepare for the child's transfer into a regular school.*

Both techniques also stress multi-sensory learning; that is, learning achieved by channeling the stimulus through the different senses.

Some concrete suggestions for language therapy are as follows:

1. *Concrete Language*
    a. *Receptive language*—parts of the body (animals, members of the family, etc.) are fairly concrete terms and may be used to initiate such therapy. Present pictures, toys, and if possible, the actual object and attempt to

---

* Mildred McGinnis has recently had published *Aphasic Children*, Alexander Graham Bell Assoc. for the Deaf, 1963.

relate the symbol to the stimulus. Relate this phase of the program to other phases of the program by using word symbols containing sounds taught in perceptual training. Also try to develop concepts by using related terms, e.g., parts of the body, etc.

b. *Expressive language*—through various speech activities ask the child to say the word symbols you have previously worked with. Do not, at this stage, be overly anxious about his articulation.

2. *Abstract Language*

After a firm base of approximately seventy-five to one hundred concrete words has been developed, the therapist can initiate work on more abstract symbols, e.g., numbers ("Give me five pennies"—the symbol "five" is abstract since it can and does refer to five of anything), up-down, etc.

3. *Phonemic-retention Training*

The following techniques may be used in phonemic training. Both articulation and language are enhanced as a result of such training. Prepare phoneme cards, with each card being of a distinctive color. Teach the child six or seven consonants followed by the vowels. The child may feel or trace the letter. For added clues, each phoneme has an individual gesture, e.g., M is characterized by placing the finger at the side of the mouth.

After approximately six or seven consonants have been learned, the therapist begins teaching the vowels beginning with *a-e*. The vowel cards should be made with black foregrounds on grey backgrounds. When the children are able to recognize most of the vowels and consonants, they should be taught to blend them into simple words which are used (whenever possible) during the receptive-expressive language training time.

4. *Mowrer's autistic theory of language development* stresses rewards in the form of acceptance, praise, etc. *before* each therapy situation is initiated.

5. *The Parsons Project in Language and Communication* (Kansas) has studied verbal behavior as a response

sequence between two persons, and failures in verbal learning by the child are evaluated in terms of the behavior of both the child and the other person. Implicit in this concept is the alteration of the listeners response; that is, exploring different reward type situations (11).

Neuromuscular Training for Neuromotor Deficiencies

There are at least five well-recognized neuromuscular re-education techniques. To be successful in the administration of these techniques requires specialized training.

A. *The Phelps Method*—Phelps utilizes the technique of "confusion motion" for muscle re-education. Confusion motion occurs in one part of the body when another part of the body is moved. For example, a child who cannot tighten his lips voluntarily will often be able to do so when asked to bite a block between his teeth. Another child who has difficulty in raising the tongue tip can often perform this movement when the therapist attempts to hold the mouth open while the child tries to close his mouth. This type of movement has been labeled "confusion motion" because there is no relationship between the confused motion and the intended motion.

Confusion motions are brought under voluntary control by the following: (1) the motion is induced repeatedly by resisting the "willed motion," (i.e., closing the mouth), (2) resistance is gradually reduced until the motion becomes voluntary.

B. *Kabat Method of Resistive Therapy*—Speech is the most complex function of any that our muscles are called upon to perform. Some of the muscles which allow for speech are also involved in more basic activities such as respiration, deglutition, etc. It follows, therefore, that the more efficiently the musculature can be developed or trained to serve the basic functions, the more ready it will be for speech development. The earlier this development occurs, the better the chances of developing speech readiness.

Basic to this treatment technique is active resistance by the therapist to the patient's innate functions, such as breathing. We know that the child is going to continue breathing and if we offer resistance, he will exert some effort to overcome the resistance. Resistance to respiration can be applied by crossing the child's elbows over his chest with some simultaneous downward pressure, timing it with an exhalation. Reduce the resistance gradually, making him work fairly hard at the beginning of the inhalation, then helping him on to a good deep breath by carrying the motion of his arms on to full extension of the rib cage.

C. *The Temple Fay Method*—This method is primarily concerned with re-education of gross (or primitive) movements of the trunk and extremities, as opposed to re-education of fine muscle actions as utilized in speech. The treatment is administered in sand or water.

D. *The Deaver Method*—The Deaver Method emphasizes the importance of training with the "activities of daily living" constantly in mind. The patient is trained by the therapist to turn door knobs, operate light switches, step up and down curbs, as well as in activities of dressing, feeding and other forms of self care.

E. *The Bobath Method*—The Bobaths devised their technique in hope of inhibiting hypertonicity. When the patient is placed in certain positions (reflex-inhibiting postures) it was found that the hypertonus decreased. It is during this period of "normalcy" that muscular habilitation is initiated. These periods of "normalcy" are attained by using some fifty reflex-inhibiting postures designed by the Bobaths. Each child is carefully studied for abnormal postures in the prone, supine, kneeling, sitting, standing, and walking positions.

One or more of these neuromuscular training techniques is usually used with the cerebral palsied child. The prime functions of the physical therapist (and sometimes corrective therapist) are muscle analysis and re-education (primarily involving the legs); therefore, the physical therapist usually masters these neuromuscular training techniques. It is not uncommon, however, for the occupational therapist or speech therapist to make use of these techniques in their training programs. The latter being primarily concerned, of course, with the speech activities of the child while the former, the occupational therapist, is mainly concerned with activities of daily living involving chiefly the upper extremities and the mechanics of grasp, release, and placement, with its subsequent application to feeding, dressing, and pre-writing skills.

BEHAVIORAL PROBLEMS AND THEIR HABILITATION

There are many behavioral abnormalities that may be seen in this type child (particularly the brain-damaged child). Some of them are: distractibility, hyper-activity, catastrophic mood changes, disinhibition, ego-centricity, and perseveration. Possible therapy for these problems is as follows:

1. *Distractibility*—this problem is caused by the presence of environmental stimuli which causes a short attention span. Therapy, therefore, should entail procedures by which the child can learn to "tune-out" to unwanted stimuli and "tune-in" to the desired stimulus. The former can be achieved by creating a "barren" environment, free of unwanted stimuli, and *gradually* exposing him to these influences. Conversely, one can also be teaching him, at the same time, to pay more attention to that which is desirable by using puzzles of appropriate difficulty. Such tasks usually motivate attention and also develop the perceptual ability to "see relationships among parts" and to "see the whole" composed of many parts.

2. *Hyperactivity*—this characteristic is perhaps the most annoying to parents. Tranquilizers, as well as education, can help to attentuate the problem. Many times it is diffi-

cult to find the appropriate tranquilizer and/or the correct dosage, but once found it proves to be of unestimable value.* By education, it is meant that one sets "limits" and constantly reminds the child what behavior is acceptable or unacceptable.

3. *Catastrophic Mood Changes*—there are three ways of handling this problem: (1) distract the child; (2) ignore the child; (3) try to stop the behavior. These mood changes, however, are usually caused by undue frustrations, and as previously pointed out, the child has a low tolerance level to stress situations and hence is easily frustrated. Try to control his environment.

4. *Disinhibition*—due to an inability to inhibit his feelings, the child gives vent, immediately, to his urges and desires. The therapist, therefore, should not tell the child that some *future* event will take place since the feelings felt by the child will be immediately expressed. As in catastrophic mood changes, the therapist can distract the child or follow any of the other suggestions.

5. *Egocentricity*—the world revolves around the child (as the child sees it) and he feels personally involved in all situations. One can point out to him (while accepting his feelings) that other children are also involved in this situation.

6. *Perseveration*—the child who continues to produce a given response when it is no longer appropriate is manifesting perseveration. These responses can best be handled by distracting him to another task requiring a completely different response. If possible, however, first present a situation in which the perseverated response will become a *correct* response and *then* change the activity to something quite different.

———————

* Some tranquilizers make the child more hyperactive, some have no discernable effect, and some make the child so tranquil that it appears as if he is in a "dream state." Only usage allows one to determine what effect a particular drug and particular dosage will have on a child.

MUSIC THERAPY

As with art and play therapies, music therapy allows for communication when other means of communicating are impaired. It is also beneficial because it influences attitudes and moods, develops attention span, and attenuates hyperactivity and distractability. It is also a useful technique in developing perceptual-motor abilities and auditory discrimination abilities. There is a national organization of music therapists; people who are particularly trained to make use of music in a therapy program.

Dance

Simple dance movements which involve pulling and pushing with two hands, in contrast to activities involving working and supporting with the hands, may be useful as exercises and coordinated movement techniques. For example, the children may be asked to sit in a chair or on the floor. They can perform the movements of rowing a boat to the tune of "Row, Row, Row Your Boat." Through the push and pull action, they develop a more coordinated use of hands and arms.

Another type of dance activity which can be used beneficially is one in which whole body patterns are involved. The weight of the body is borne partially or fully by different parts of the body. The purpose of such an activity would be to further enrich awareness of symmetry and asymmetry. For example, creeping on all fours in the pretense of being jungle animals to the tune of "Chicken-Licken." This causes all four limbs to carry weight in a successive, reciprocal manner.

Exercises to develop awareness of the relationship of the joints, and folding, and unfolding of the limbs can be brought forth by the use of the somersault and supported headstands and handstands. By the somersault, the child experiences rotation through space. By headstands and handstands, the child can experience the distribution of weight. It might be noted that these techniques should be used with care, for many children fear being turned upside down in such an unfamiliar spatial relationship. The child should be primed and coached for such an experience. Each type of exercise is performed to the accompaniment of such music as "Elfin Dance."

Vocal Activities

Children of all types, "normal" or "abnormal," generally love to sing in one fashion or another. Thus, for the brain-damaged the enjoyment of vocalizing would seem to be just as prevalent as in the normal child. If language has developed or is being taught to the brain-damaged child, simple songs such as "Mary Had A Little Lamb," or "Hickory Dickory Dock" can be taught. The therapist repeats the words several times and then sings the song for the children. If the therapist puts enough expression into the song the children will, in most cases, be eager to try singing the song when they are asked. If the children do not have sufficient language, they can always take the part of a fire engine, a train, or small animal in a song which appropriately calls for such noises. For example, "Down by the Station" calls for the "toot-toot," "woo-woo" of a train. "Old McDonald Had A Farm" calls for various animal sounds.

It can be seen that different types of vocal activities can be employed to suit the ability of the child. If songs are taught, however, and the child cannot actually retain the words or correctly use them, he should not be stopped if he hums along or tries to carry the tune by means of grunts or jabbering sounds. As long as he participates, much is being accomplished in the way of cutting down on hyperactivity and in increasing his attention span. If the child has language, but is handicapped by an extremely short attention span, use of the same songs may help to increase his attention span as the child becomes familiar with the words. The therapist must always be ready to vary the program, however, when signs of renewed hyperactivity and short attention span begin to appear.

Rhythmical Activity

Almost invariably, a child responds to rhythm, which is music's most dynamic component. Non-verbal children have the same needs, desires, and aggressions as do other children, even though they lack normal means of expression. By means of rhythm instruments, the therapist provides a means of combining social adaptation with muscular control and increased attention span. At first, these children usually bang at random; but they learn to control their energies according to the requirements of the music. In the formation of a rhythm band, the aggressive can beat drums and symbols, and the more timid may begin with "gentle" instruments such as triangles and bells. The choice of instruments should be left to the children as much as possible so as to strengthen their initiative. Their choice is often a good clue to their personality and self-image. When a timid child, after playing in the rhythm band for awhile, comes forth and chooses an aggressive instrument such as the drum, it is a significant gesture as to a possible change in the child's self concept. The same applies if an aggressive child should choose a "gentle" instrument.

ART THERAPY

All children, in varying degrees, can "express" themselves through the medium of color, paint, muscular action of finger painting, and clay pounding. Because the "unusual child" may be retarded in other means of expression, art may be his only way to interact with his society—his only way (or another way) of communicating with his environment. Many times, through art, the child is able to communicate to others his reactions to life situations which he encounters in his environment, whether it be in the home, in the school, or in the community.

The therapist or parent can also gain insight into what the child does not understand about himself or his environment through art activities. For example, after a trip to the zoo the child is asked to draw a picture of what he has seen. The child might leave the bars off the cage implying that he missed the idea of the animals being locked up. The parent or therapist would then know what points are to be emphasized on future trips to the zoo.

Art experiences also bring to light instabilities, emotional conflicts and insecurities. Through special activities such as finger painting and clay modeling, many fears and dislikes are released through aggressive behavior. When the child is able to express his feelings about a fear, the fear is often attenuated through this expression.

Because the child has experienced many failures and set-backs in his life, he often needs a boost in self-confidence. Through art he may acquire this self-confidence and enhance his self-concept. It is then quite possible that he will participate more freely in other activities. The child must achieve success if he is to actively grow in social and personal development.

Social control is another benefit gained from art activities. Through art activities the youngster learns to relate to other people and adjust to a social group.

Art activities also help develop perceptual abilities. As the mentally handicapped child scribbles or handles lumps of clay, he gains greater kinesthetic and tactile awareness. As he paints or draws, he responds to color and form, thus growing in visual awareness. Art work also allows for development of hand-eye coordination.

Development of Artistic Expression

The developmental process of artistic expression in the "unusual child" follows basically the same pattern as that of the normal child but may be much slower.

Gaitskell (6) breaks the artistic development into four stages. The first of which is the manipulative stage. This is the experimental scribbling period in which random marks and forms are utilized. The mentally subnormal child, for example, may remain in this stage for as long as three years before progressing to the second stage. Because the retardate usually remains in this stage a long period of time, he often learns to coordinate his hands better than the normal child.

The second stage is related to symbolization. The child begins to place symbols in his work that resemble objects in his world of experience. The first symbol is usually a human being. Development of these symbols may progress to include abstract concepts before the child moves into the next stage. There is no set time limit for each stage, as each child is different in this developmental process.

After placing the objects in the picture, the child then places these objects within a pictorial setting; this is the schematic stage. The child now uses sky, grass, trees, and other accessories in this work.

In this schematic phase of development there are three techniques utilized with the "unusual child" that are not frequently found in the work of the normal child. They include the x-ray picture, the fold-over picture, and the series picture. The x-ray picture makes it possible for the child to see what's inside, e.g., a school showing the outside and the pupils inside. The fold-over picture requires the folding of the paper to place the objects in correct perspective. Both the x-ray and the fold-over picture represent the difficulty the child encounters with the problem of perspective. The third is the series picture which connects objects of similar thought.

The fourth stage of development is realism. In this phase the child begins to solve the problem of perspective, to use better color and background and to overlap objects. This stage is sometimes never reached by the normal child as well as the mentally retarded.

Art Activities

Puppetry is recommended as an appropriate group activity. The children should design their own puppets (can be made from paper bags) and learn to move the fold of the bag in synchronization with spoken lines, possibly from a well-liked story or some experience. They receive enjoyment from this activity and grow in expression and social control at the same time.

Mural making is another good group activity. This activity requires a plan and discussion by the group; then each child works independently on one thing.

Group activities can be difficult, however, and sometime present problems in class control. Individual activities are often better, especially in the earlier stages of development. Popular individual activities include finger painting, clay modeling, and drawing.

Suitable Materials

Wax crayons of good quality are considered to be the best all-purpose medium. The child should be taught to color freely and with considerable pressure.

Tempera paint is practical if supplied in separate jars of red, yellow, blue, green, brown, black, and white. Also needed are brushes of good quality. This material should not be used by very young children since many materials in use at one time tend to confuse them.

Paper for drawing and painting should be large and heavy because of the many corrections the retardate will make. Sheets of paper should be big and should be of neutral color. Manila paper is the most acceptable.

Construction paper, gold and silver paper, scraps of wall paper, corrugated paper, or sand paper can be used for cutting and pasting. Other materials with texture are excellent for this purpose.

Additional materials that should be available are individual tables and chairs that are movable, running hot and cold water, large display boards, and labeled storage places for each child's work.

PLAY THERAPY

Moustakas (10) mentions six levels of normal emotional growth:

A. *First level*—characterized by undifferentiated and ill-defined positive and negative feelings.
B. *Second level*—characterized by the emergence of focused positive and negative feelings in response to parents, siblings, and other people in the environment.
C. *Third level*—characterized by ambivalent feelings.
D. *Fourth level*—characterized by negative feelings in primary focus.
E. *Fifth level*—characterized by negative and positive attitudes that are ambivalent.

F. *Sixth level*—characterized by predominantly positive attitudes which appear as organized attitudes; negative attitudes are also present but they are in line with reality.

Play therapy is needed when a child is unable to make the step to the next level of growth.

Play therapy, however, is not only used for disturbed children, but often for all children in a mental hygiene program. Every child can benefit when given an opportunity to express himself. All children have frustrating experiences which they cannot express at home or school.

What is Play Therapy

Play therapy may be directive or non-directive. Today, non-directive therapy in the play situation is used almost exclusively.

Non-directive play therapy is based on the assumption that the individual has within himself, not only the ability to solve his own problems satisfactorily, but also the growth impulse that makes mature behavior more satisfying than immature behavior. The child has the opportunity to grow under the most favorable conditions. By playing out his feelings of tension, frustration, insecurity, aggression, fear, bewilderment, and confusion; he learns to face them, control them, or abandon them.

There are three basic attitudes in child-centered play therapy; they are, faith, acceptance, and respect. The therapist must convey these attitudes.

Faith is intangible, and yet in the presence of another person who has faith in us, we are able to grasp that feeling and are able to face ourselves, to grow within ourselves and to create more of ourselves. The child senses that the therapist has faith in him. This becomes reflected in the child when he considers himself to be an important person. He is able to make decisions and carry them out. He is able to freely express himself without fear. In order for the therapist to express faith in the child, he must truly have faith in the child—a belief that children have within themselves the capacity for self-growth and self-realization.

In acceptance, the therapist is more passive. He accepts the child's feelings and his personal meanings.

Objects convey different meanings to different children. Sand, clay, water, or another object may symbolize a parent, a sibling, a particular fear, or almost anything. The therapist must accept the child's symbolism as it is. Words will not convey acceptance unless the therapist actually feels this acceptance. The therapist should neither disapprove and criticize, nor approve and reward; for example, if the therapist rewards the child's behavior, the child may limit himself to only those actions which bring approval by the therapist.

Respect is closely allied to faith and acceptance. If the child feels respected, he feels that his interests and feelings are understood. This relationship can be developed in patient-clinician interactions. Respect goes a step beyond acceptance; it indicates to the child that he is regarded as worthwhile and important.

These three attitudes—faith, acceptance, and respect are basic to success in play therapy.

Contrary to the belief of some individuals, play therapy does not mean that the therapist merely sits with the child for an hour while he plays; but it is a process in which definite principles must be observed. Axline (3) lists the principles as follows:

A. The therapist must develop a warm, friendly relationship with the child in which good rapport is established as soon as possible. This is done through acceptance of the child as he is from the very beginning of the therapy program.

B. The therapist accepts the child exactly as he is. (This is merely a continuation of the preceeding principle.) The therapist is calm, steady, and friendly; he avoids praise and reproof. Acceptance does not mean approval of what the child does; nor does it mean suggesting to the child what to do.

C. The therapist establishes a feeling of permissiveness in the relationship so that the child feels free to express his feelings completely. The hour belongs to the child and he should be able to use it in any way he likes. The child should have the choice of which toys to use. Complete lack of suggestion is conducive to successful therapy.

D. The therapist is able to recognize the feelings the child is expressing and reflect back those feelings in such a manner that the child gains insight into his own behavior. If the child asks a factual question, it is advisable to answer it directly. Recognition and interpretation of feelings are two different things. The child's play is symbolic of his feelings and when the therapist attempts to translate this behavior into words, he says what he thinks the child feels. At times, interpretation is unavoidable, but it should be used very cautiously.

E. The therapist maintains a deep respect for the child's ability to solve his own problems if given an opportunity. The responsibility to make choices and institute change is the child's. He needs to achieve independence, self confidence, and self respect.

F. The therapist does not attempt to direct the child's actions or conversation in any manner. The child leads the way, the therapist follows. The therapist offers no suggestions. If the child asks for directions as to how to use the materials, the clinician should furnish the information.

G. The therapist does not attempt to hurry the therapy along. It is a gradual process and should be recognized as such by the therapist. When the child is ready, he will express his feelings, but he cannot be hurried. Too often, at home, the child is not allowed to do anything for himself because he "takes all day."

H. The therapist establishes only those limitations that are necessary to anchor therapy to the world of reality and to make the child aware of his responsibility in the relationship. A limitation on time, self-harm, and harm to the therapist should be set. Axline feels that limitations should not be imposed until the need arises.

The therapeutic process follows a regular pattern. At first, the child's emotions are diffuse and undifferentiated and mostly negative. The child may be frightened, angry, or immature without definitely focusing his feelings on any particular person; he seems afraid of almost everything and everybody. As the relationship between the child and the therapist is clarified, the hostility becomes more specific. Anger is often related to particular persons. The child may threaten the therapist, a parent, a sibling, or an entire family. As feelings are accepted, they become less intense.

At the third level, the child is no longer completely negative in his responses and expressions of feelings. He may still be angry, but often he is ambivalent in his feelings toward people.

In the final stage, positive feelings begin to emerge. He now sees himself and his relationships with people more realistically.

These steps are not clearly definable and are often overlapping.

What Materials Should the Play Room Contain

The play therapy room itself should be sound proof, if possible, and contain a sink with hot and cold running water. The walls and floors should be constructed of material that is easily cleaned.

Play materials should include nursing bottles, doll family, doll house and furniture, toy soldiers, army equipment, toy animals, dishes, pans, spoons, doll clothes, clothespins, clothes basket, large rag doll, puppets, puppet screen, crayons, clay, finger paints, sand, water, toy guns, peg pounding sets, wooden mallets, paper dolls, toy cars, airplanes, table, easel, toy telephone, shelves, basin, small broom and mop, drawing paper, finger painting paper, newspapers, pictures of people, houses, animals, and other objects.

Material should be kept on shelves easily accessible to the child.

Chapter IX

CONCLUSION

W E HAVE ATTEMPTED to present a cohesive picture which will enable the reader to better understand the manifold problems of the non-verbal child.

We believe that the millions of children who present such problems are deserving of help—a multi-disciplined and intensive habilitative program—yet too frequently in our society, these children receive only fragmented help and then on a one or two hour a week basis—if they receive any treatment at all.

Such programs as we envision would necessitate a number of changes in our current practices: first, our training centers should emphasize (much more so than is currently the practice) the integrated nature of habilitation. In doing so, our therapists would, at least, be more aware of the variety of problems that beset many handicapped children. Secondly, our service centers must direct their efforts toward a total habilitative program, rather than a fragmented one. Some such facilities are already available. Many of them are operating under such a philosophy but are plagued by boards of lay-people who handicap the operation of the program because of shortsightedness; others give lip-service to the multi-discipline concept; others have ill-trained staffs.

The lead in such an effort must come from our universities. Here, the trained habilitative administrator should be granted authority to develop a training program and service center that will cater to these concepts. It should, however, be acknowledged that such a program is expensive, both in physical plant and in a highly trained diversified staff.

It is time for our society to recognize this need and help those who so frequently have no place to go for treatment.

BIBLIOGRAPHY

1. *A Proposed Program for National Action to Combat Mental Retardation: The President's Panel on Mental Retardation.* Washington: U. S. Government Printing Office, 1962, pp. 7-8.

2. Alt, H.: *Residential Treatment for the Disturbed Child: Basic Principles in Planning and Design of Programs and Facilities.* International University Press, 1961.

3. Axline, V. M.: *Play Therapy.* New York, Houghton-Mifflin Company, 1947.

4. Cannon, W. D., and Rosenbleuth, H.: *The Supersensitivity of Denervated Structures.* New York, Macmillan, 1949.

5. Eisenson, J. et al.: *The Psychology of Communication.* New York, Appleton-Century-Crofts, 1962, Chapters 12, 13.

6. Gaitskell, C. D.: *Arts and Crafts in Our Schools.* Peoria, C. A. Bennett Company, Inc., 1956.

7. Lehtinen, L. E.: The Brain-Damaged Child: What We Can Do For Him, *The Dallas Medical Journal,* 1959, pp. 15-21.

8. McCarthy, D.: Language Development in Children, (In *A Manual of Child Psychology,* Ed., L. Carmichael. 2nd Ed.) New York, Wiley, 1954, pp. 592-630.

9. Monsees, E. K.: Aphasia and Deafness in Children, *Exceptional Children, 25:*5, 1959, pp. 395-399.

10. Moustakas, C. E.: *Children in Play Therapy—A Key to Understanding Normal and Disturbed Emotions.* New York, McGraw-Hill, 1953.

11. Mowrer, O. H.: *Learning Theory and the Symbolic Process.* New York, Wiley, 1960.

12. Penfield, W., and Roberts, L.: *Speech and Brain Mechanisms.* Princeton, Princeton University Press, 1959.

13. Salmon, F.: *Rehabilitation Center Planning With Supplement.* University Park, Pennsylvania State University, 1959.

14. Schiefelbusch, R. L., et al.: Language Studies of Mentally Retarded Children, *Monograph Supplement Number Ten, Journal of Speech and Hearing Disorders,* 1963, or the Parsons Project in Language and Communication of Mentally Retarded Children, University of Kansas, Bureau of Child Research; Parsons State Hospital and Training Center.

SUGGESTED READINGS

I. General

Kephart, N. C.: *The Slow-Learner in the Classroom.* Columbus, C. E. Merrill Books, Inc., 1960.

Johnson, D. M.: *The Psychology of Thought and Judgment.* New York, Harper, 1955, pp. 102-409.

Jordon, T. E.: *The Exceptional Child.* Columbus, C. E. Merrill Books, Inc., 1962.

Roucek, J. S. (ed.): *The Unusual Child.* New York, Philosophical Library, 1962.

II. Brain Mechanism

Penfield, W., and Rasmussen, T.: *The Cerebral Cortex of Man.* New York, Macmillian, 1960.

III. The Brain Injured Child

Barry, H.: *The Young Aphasic Child: Evaluation and Training.* Washington, Alexander Graham Bell Association for the Deaf, 1961.

Cruickshank, W. M.: *Cerebral Palsy: Its Individual and Community Problems.* Syracuse, Syracuse University Press, 1955.

Hood, O. E.: *Your Child or Mine: The Brain Injured Child and His Hope.* New York, Harper, 1957.

Lewis, R. S.: *The Other Child: The Brain Injured Child, The Book for Parents and Laymen.* New York, Grune and Stratton, 1951.

Siegel, E.: *Helping the Brain Injured Child: Handbook for Parents.* New York, New York Association for Brain Injured Children, 1961.

Strauss, A., and Lehtinen, L. E.: *Psychology and Education of the Brain Injured Child* (Vol. I). New York, Grune and Stratton, 1947.

Strauss, A., and Kephart, N. C.: *Psychopathology and Education of the Brain Injured Child* (Vol. II). New York, Grune and Stratton, 1955.

110

IV. The Mentally Retarded Child

Masland, R. L.: *Mental Subnormality*: *Biological, Psychological and Cultural*. New York, Basic Books, 1959.

Rothstein, J. H.: *Mental Retardation*: *Reading and Resources*. New York, Holt, Rinehart, Winston, 1961.

V. The Emotionally Ill Child

Bower, E. M.: *Early Identification of Emotionally Handicapped Children in School*. Springfield, Thomas, 1960.

D'Evelyn, K.: *Meeting Children's Emotional Needs*. New York Prentice Hall, 1960.

VI. The Deaf Child

Myklebust, H. R.: *The Psychology of Deafness*: *Sensory Deprivation, Learning and Adjustment*. New York, Grune and Stratton, 1960.

VII. Differential Diagnosis

Brown, S. F.: The Concept of Congenital Aphasia From the Stand-Point of Dynamic Differential Diagnosis, *American Speech and Hearing Association,* 1959.

Gesell, A., and Ilg, F. L.: *The Child From Five to Ten*. New York, Harper, 1946.

Haeusserman, E.: *Developmental Potential of Preschool Children*: *An Evaluation of Intellectual, Sensory and Emotional Functioning*. New York, Grune and Stratton, 1958.

Montague, A.: *Pre-Natal Influences*. Springfield, Thomas, 1962.

Myklebust, H. R.: *Auditory Disorders in Children*: *A Manual for Differential Diagnosis*. New York, Grune and Stratton, 1954.

Strean, L. P.: *The Normal Birth of Normal Babies*. New York, Twayne, 1958.

Wood, N. E., "Decision Making: Childhood Aphasia, *ASHA,* April 1962, pp. 571-575.

VIII. Habilitation

1. *Hearing Therapy*

   Davis, H., and Silverman, S. R.: *Hearing and Deafness* (Rev. Ed.). New York, Holt, Rinehart, 1960.

   Lassman, G. H.: *Language for the Preschool Deaf Child*. New York, Grune and Stratton, 1950.

   Whitehurst, M. W.: *Auditory Training Manual*. New York, Hearing Rehabilitation Center, 1949.

2. *Language Therapy*

  Travis, L. E. (ed.): *Handbook of Speech Pathology*. New York,
  Appleton-Century-Crofts, Inc., 1957, Selected Chapters.

3. *Neuromuscular Therapy*

  Abbot, M.: *A Syllabus of Cerebral Palsy Treatment Techniques*.
  Iowa, William C. Brown, 1957.

4. *Music Therapy*

  National Association for Music Therapy, *Music Therapy: Book of
  Proceedings*, Vol. I. through VIII. Lawrence, Kansas, National
  Association for Music Therapy, 1956-1958.

5. *Art Therapy*

  Gaitskell, C., and Gaitskell, M.: *Art Expression for Slow Learners*.
  Peoria, C. A. Bennett Company, Inc., 1953.

  Lowenfeld, V.: *Your Child and His Art*. New York, Macmillian
  Company, 1955.

6. *Psychotherapy*

  Ginott, H. G.: *Group Psychotherapy With Children: The Theory
  and Practice of Play Therapy*. New York, McGraw-Hill, 1961.

APPENDIX I

Sample Forms Used To Collect Case-History Data

EAST TENNESSEE STATE UNIVERSITY
COLLEGE OF HEALTH
SPEECH AND HEARING CLINIC

CONFIDENTIAL MEDICAL REPORT—MAIL TO CLINIC

Name of Patient................................Age.......Birth-Date.............Sex........

Patient's Address................................Parent's Name.........................

Examined by................................GP......PED......ENT......Neuro......Other......

Examiner's Address................................

Complaint: 1. Stuttering ☐   2. Articulation ☐   3. Voice ☐
           4. Language ☐   5. Hearing ☐   6. Other.................

Is speech or hearing therapy contraindicated?........................

	Normal	*Abnormal*	*Comment*
Eyes	....	....	....
Ears	....	....	....
Tongue	....	....	....
Lingual Frenum	....	....	....
Lips	....	....	....
Tonsils & Adenoids	....	....	....
Hard Palate	....	....	....
Soft Palate	....	....	....
Uvula	....	....	....

Were there any indications of the following:
    Crainal Nerve Damage   ☐ Yes ( ) ☐ No ( ) ☐ (?)
    Central Nervous System Damage ☐ Yes ( ) ☐ No ( ) ☐ (?)
    Mental Retardation   ☐ Yes ( ) ☐ No ( ) ☐ (?)
    Emotional Disorder   ☐ Yes ( ) ☐ No ( ) ☐ (?)

Is the patient currently receiving treatment?   ☐ Yes ☐ No

If yes, what is the nature of this treatment?................................
....

Is there any additional information which might be of help?........................
....
....

....
Signature of Physician

Would like a copy of our examination report ☐

113

EAST TENNESSEE STATE UNIVERSITY
COLLEGE OF HEALTH
SPEECH AND HEARING CLINIC

CONFIDENTIAL REPORT—TO BE MAILED TO CLINIC

TO THE TEACHER OR PRINCIPAL: In order that we may have more information about this child, we ask you to complete this form and return it to the clinic.

EDUCATIONAL HISTORY

Name ....Grade......Birth Date................. Date................

Name of School..Address..

I.   Achievement in School Subjects

     A.   Elementary   B.   High School

	Poor	Average	Good		Poor	Average	Good
Reading	....	....	....	English	....	....	....
Spelling	....	....	....	Math	....	....	....
Arithmetic	....	....	....	Science	....	....	....
Writing	....	....	....	Foreign Lang.	....	....	....
Language	....	....	....	Industrial Arts	....	....	....
Art	....	....	....	Social	....	....	....
Citizenship	....	....	....	Other Subjects	....	....	....

Comments: ....
....
....

II.   Tests that have been administered at school:

     Intelligence: Name of................C.A.....M.A.....I.Q.....When administered........

                       Name of................C.A.....M.A.....I.Q.....When administered........

     Achievement: Name of..........................When administered..............................

                 What is his grade level of achievement?...................................

III.   Behavior ....
....

     Please provide below, or on the back of this page, additional information which might be of help to the speech and hearing clinic.

....
                                 Signature of Principal or Teacher

Would like copy of East Tennessee State University Evaluation. ☐

EAST TENNESSEE STATE UNIVERSITY
COLLEGE OF HEALTH
SPEECH AND HEARING CLINIC

Patient's Name...Age.........Birth Date...................

Speech and/or Hearing Problem...

....

TO THE PARENT: Following is a list of common childhood problems. Indicate if your child has such a problem. Bring this form with you when you come to the clinic for the examination.

	Problem	No Problem
Nervousness	....	....
Sleeplessness	....	....
Nightmares	....	....
Bed wetting	....	....
Playing with sex organs	....	....
Walking in sleep	....	....
Shyness	....	....
Showing off	....	....
Refusal to obey	....	....
Rudeness	....	....
Fighting	....	....
Selfishness	....	....
Lying	....	....
Tongue sucking	....	....
Hurting pets	....	....
Setting fires	....	....
Constipation	....	....
Thumb sucking	....	....
Face twitching	....	....
Fainting	....	....
Strong fears	....	....
Strong hates	....	....
Queer food habits	....	....
Running away	....	....
Temper tantrums	....	....
Whining	....	....
Stealing	....	....
Destructiveness	....	....
Others...........................	....	....

Developmental History

At what approximate age was your child able to do the following? Place a check on the appropriate line if you think he was early, normal, or late in doing these things.

		Approximate Age	Early	Normal	Late
1.	Roll over°	....	....	....	....
2.	Sit unsupported	....	....	....	....
3.	Stand alone	....	....	....	....
1.	Walk unattended	....	....	....	....
2.	Pull off his socks	....	....	....	....
3.	Drink from a cup or glass unassisted	....	....	....	....
4.	Eat with a spoon	....	....	....	....
5.	Talk in short sentences	....	....	....	....
1.	Eat with a fork	....	....	....	....
2.	Put on—take off coat	....	....	....	....
3.	Ask to go to the toilet	....	....	....	....
1.	Button his coat (or dress, etc.)	....	....	....	....
2.	Wash his hands unaided	....	....	....	....
3.	Walk downstairs one step per tread	....	....	....	....

° The numbering is arranged so that one can tell at a glance if the child was early, normal, or late in his development. The first group (1, 2, 3) of activities should be performed within the first year; the second group (1, 2, 3, 4, 5) within the second year and so on. This information does not appear on the form that is sent to the parent.

EAST TENNESSEE STATE UNIVERSITY
COLLEGE OF HEALTH
SPEECH AND HEARING CLINIC

GENERAL CASE HISTORY

I. *Identifying Information*:

Name of Patient...Birth Date.........................Age............

Address .... Telephone...............................

Father's Name...Occupation.................................

Education .... Age..............

Mother's Name...Occupation..................................

Education .... Age..............

How many children (other than patient) do you have, their ages, and do they have any problems (s & h, behavior, or educational); e.g., Mary 12, o.k.

....

....

Is anyone else living in the home, if so, what is the relationship; does their presence affect the family in any way?...

....

History taken by...Informant.....................................

Date of Examination..........................Referred by.......................................

II. *Problem*:
Informant's description of problem..
....

Any similar problems in family (other than siblings), and if so, what is this
person's degree of contact with patient. Describe relationship...............................
....
.... ,..

III. *Pre-Natal History*: (If significant, go into detail)
Illnesses (when)...
Physical Health...
Emotional Health..
    (1) Were any medicines (especially for tension) taken during the pregnancy?
       If so, name of drug and why taken...
       ....

    (2) How did you and your husband feel when you knew you were going to
       have a baby? (Was informant upset, was baby unplanned or unwanted?)
       ....

    (3) Was the pregnancy a pleasant and happy period?...................If not, why?
       (Was there any marital discord, did parents "fuss" a lot?).........................
       ....

False labor (when and under what conditions)..
History of miscarriages..
Other unusual conditions (falls, blows, Rh incompatibility)....................................
Were you treated by a doctor during the pregnancy for anything unusual? If yes,
describe nature and purpose of treatment...
....

IV. *Birth History*:
Term of Pregnancy (try to be exact)..
How much time elapsed between the first indication of labor and the delivery?
....

Birth Weight...
Type of birth:
a. Normal.....................
b. Breech....................... Comments...
c. Cesarean................... Why..
d. Abnormalities during presentation...
    1. Dry birth (if so, when did the water (amniotic sac) break, how long
       before delivery)..
    2. Cord strangulation ....
    3. Delayed breathing (how soon after delivery did he cry?)...........................
    4. Other ....

V. *Immediate Post-Natal History*: (If significant, go into detail)
Scars, bruises or deformities at birth (especially of head)......................................
....

Seizures or convulsions (does he ever stare as if in a trance—is this behavior
habitual etc., look for evidence of Jacksonian, petite-mal or grand-mal types of
epilepsy) ....
Feeding difficulties..

Breathing difficulties..
Skin Hue Blue (anoxic) ....
            Yellow (Jaundice) ....
Did baby cry a lot (colic)—did it cause parents much trouble (was it a fretful
baby as opposed to a good baby?)...
General Health of baby...

VI. *Post-Natal History*: (If significant, go into detail)
1. Was he slow in his development, e.g., walking, etc.?.....................................

    ----
2. Was he awkward or clumsy?...
3. Is he a "slow" child in general?..

VII. *Child-Rearing Philosophy*: (If significant, go into detail)
What means do you use to discipline your child?...

Is there a lot of fussing-bickering between mother—child; father—child?...............

Do you and your husband (or wife) disagree as to child rearing practices?
(What is nature of husband-wife relationship—are they compatible?)....................

VIII. *History of Illness*: (If significant, go into detail)
1. Was there any difference in the patient's behavior after an illness as compared
    to his behavior before the illness?...
2. Has patient had persistent trouble with ears?..

IX. *Surgery*:
T & A (when, by whom, and why)..
Other (when, by whom, and why)..

X. *Behavioral Adjustment*: (If significant, go into detail)
Is the child extremely (as compared to other children his age):
1. Hyperactive—is he always on the go—does he seem to have a surplus of energy?

    ----
2. Distractible—is he constantly exploring his environment—looking, listening
    and touching?..
3. Withdrawn, shy, timid...
4. Aggressive ....
5. Impulsive—is he often unable to control his impulses, and therefore ("blows
    his top") reacts emotionally?..
6. Perseverative—does he find it difficult to shift from one situation to another—
    does he continue to respond when the stimulus for such a response is no
    longer there (e.g., continue to pound a nail after it has gone all the way into
    the wood)?..
7. Peculiar in way he laughs or crys—if so, give details:...................................
8. Did he have extremely long periods of crying when he was an infant? If so,
    give details:...

    ----
9. Other ....

XI. *Auditory Behavior*: (If significant, go into detail)
Does your child:

1. Seem to ignore sound willfully (or is he inconsistent in his hearing behavior?)
    ....
2. Have difficulty hearing you?..
3. Have difficulty hearing his teacher?..
4. Raise volume of the T.V. or radio unusually loud?..
XII. *Previous therapy*........................ If yes, answer the following:
1. Who gave it?..
2. When and how long?..
3. Where? ....
4. What was done?..
XIII. *TO THE STUDENT CLINICIAN:*
1. On the basis of the case-history data you have just obtained, as well as the educational, developmental, behavioral, and medical data previously discussed, what is your:
    a. diagnosis
    b. etiology
2. If the etiology (above) is cerebral dysfunction, what are the specific areas of dysfunction?
3. If the etiology (above) is functional, what is the specific functional cause(s) of this disorder?
4. What is the parents' attitude toward the condition and the correction of the condition?
5. How much parental cooperation can we expect re: their attitudes and educational backgrounds?
6. Compatibility and general well-being of family:
    a. Harmony or discord..
    b. Unusual disease conditions..
    c. Unusual physical conditions..
    d. Etc. ....
7. Is there any indication of emotional mal-adjustment and if so, what implications does it have in terms of the speech therapy program?

APPENDIX II

Case-History and Progress Report on a Nine Year Old Minimally Brain-injured Child. This Child Was Seen Five Days a Week During the Summer of 1962. During this Time She Received Speech Therapy, Special Education, and Remedial Reading Therapy Each Day

Patient's Address:
February 3, 1962

Dr. Sol Adler
East Tennessee State College
Johnson City, Tennessee
Dear Dr. Adler:

For some time I have been looking for a good speech clinic, and just recently heard of yours through one of the professors here. I would like a diagnosis, and possible treatment, for my daughter, age nine. She has had short terms of therapy under three different teachers, but they do not live here, and it was so hard to reach them, we failed to keep going.

Since I teach, and my daughter is in school, I'm wondering if you could give us an appointment for some Saturday. Also, will you give me some information as to the treatment, should you feel you can help her. Do you hold classes, or work privately with each student? How long per day or any other information you think I might need to know? Of course, I realize that you can tell me more after seeing her.

I shall appreciate an early reply.

Very sincerely yours,

February 8 1962

Parent's Name
Address

Dear——————:

We shall be very happy to see your daughter on Saturday, February 17, 1962 at 10:00.

In answer to your questions: we work either individually and/or in groups with the children, depending upon their needs. We usually see our patients one or two times a week with sessions lasting for about one hour.

We shall be happy, however, to discuss these and other questions with you at the time of your appointment.

Enclosed you will find a medical referral form for her doctor to fill out, an educational history form for her teacher to complete and a developmental history form for you to fill out. Please return them to us by mail or bring them with you when you come to the clinic. It is important that we have these forms before we examine your child.

The Speech and Hearing Clinic is located on the second floor of the Health Building, room 208.

If you are unable to keep this appointment, please write to us or call us at WAlnut 6-1112, Ext. 272.

Sincerely,

Sol Adler, Ph.D., Director
Speech and Hearing Clinic

SA:jmp

SPEECH AND HEARING CLINIC
DEPARTMENT OF HEALTH EDUCATION
EAST TENNESSEE STATE COLLEGE*

WAlnut 6-1112, Ext. 272

MEDICAL REFERRAL FORM

Name of Patient _____ Age Nine Sex Female

Patient's Address _____ Parent's Name _____

Examined by M.D. ☐ GP ☒ PED ☐ ENT ☐ Neuro ☐ Other ☒ Cardiology

Examiner's Address _____

Would you like to receive a report of our diagnosis/evaluation? ☒ Yes ☐ No

COMPLAINT: 1. Stuttering ☐   2. Articulation ☒   3. Voice ☒
           4. Language ☐   5. Hearing ☐   6. Other ☐

Is speech or hearing therapy contraindicated? ___No___

	Normal	Abnormal	Comments
Eyes	X		
Ears	X		
Tongue	X		
Lingual Frenum	X		
Lips	X		
Tonsils and Adenoids	X	Enucleated	
Hard Palate	X		
Soft Palate	X		
Uvula	X		

Were there any indications of the following:

Cranial nerve damage   ☐ Yes   ☐ No   ☐ (?)

Central nervous system damage   ☒ Yes   ☐ No   ☐ (?)

Mental retardation   ☐ Yes   ☒ No   ☐ (?)

Is the patient currently receiving treatment?   ☐ Yes   ☒ No

If yes, what is the nature of this treatment?

Is there any additional information which might be of help?   Patient had
intracranial hemorrhage at birth.

M.D.
Signature of Physician

---

* ETSC was subsequently granted university status. This form and others that follow are now outmoded and those previously presented are in current use at our clinic.

SPEECH AND HEARING CLINIC
DEPARTMENT OF HEALTH EDUCATION
EAST TENNESSEE STATE COLLEGE

TO THE TEACHER OR PRINCIPAL: In order that we may have complete information about this child, we ask you to complete this form and return it to the clinic.

EDUCATIONAL HISTORY

Name _____ Grade 3 Date of Birth 12/16/52 Date 2/15/62

Name of School _____ Address _____

I. Achievement in School Subjects
   A. Elementary   B. High School

	Poor	Average	Good			Poor	Average	Good
Reading	X			English				
Spelling	X			Math				
Arithmetic		X		Science				
Writing	X			Social Studies				
Language	X			Foreign Lang.				
Art		X		Industrial Arts				
Citizenship			X	Other subjects				

Comments   The above refers not to failures, but most of her work is below average. Subject failed reading for the term this year.

II. Tests that have been administered at school.

Intelligence:

Name of Calif. M.M. C.A.   M.A.   I.Q. 98 When administered 3/29/60

Name of Otis AS C.A. 8.11 M.A. 7.9 I.Q. 88 When administered 11/1/61

Achievement:

Name of Calif. Achiev. X   When administered 1/18/61
What is his grade level of achievement?   2.4

III. Behavior The conduct of the subject is excellent. She has never been a problem insofar as behavior is concerned.

Please provide below or on the back of this page, additional information which might be of help to the Speech and Hearing Clinic.

The subject always puts forth a genuine effort. She is subject to forgetting what she has learned She likes school very much.

Signature of Principle or Teacher

SPEECH AND HEARING CLINIC
DEPARTMENT OF HEALTH EDUCATION
EAST TENNESSEE STATE COLLEGE

TO THE PARENT: Following is a list of common childhood problems. Check the line which indicates how often these problems occur with your child. Bring it in to the Speech and Hearing Clinic.

	Often	Seldom	Never
Nervousness		X	
Sleeplessness		X	
Nightmares			X
Bedwetting			X
Playing with sex organs			X
Walking in sleep			X
Shyness		X	
Showing off		X	
Refusal to obey		X	
Rudeness		X	
Fighting			X
Jealousy			X
Selfishness			X
Lying		X	
Smoking			X
Tongue sucking			X
Hurting pets			X
Setting fires			X
Constipation		X	
Thumb sucking			X
Face twitching			X
Fainting			X
Strong fears			X
Strong hates			X
Queer food habits		X	
Running away			X
Temper tantrums		X	
Whining		X	
Stealing			X
Destructiveness			X

Developmental History

At what approximate age was your child able to do the following. Place a check on the appropriate line if you think he was early, normal, or late in doing these things.

	Approximate Age	Early	Normal	Late
1. Roll over	3 months		X	
2. Sit unsupported	8 months		X	
3. Stand alone	1 year			X
1. Walk unattended	18 months			X
2. Pull off his socks	16 months	X		
3. Drink from a cup or glass unassisted	1 year	X		
4. Eat from a spoon	15 months	X		
5. Talk in short sentences	3 years			X
1. Eat with a fork	3 years			X
2. Put on—take off coat	3 years			X
3. Ask to go to toilet	2 years		X	
1. Button his coat (or dress, etc.)	5 years			X
2. Wash his hands unaided	3 years			X
3. Walk downstairs one step per tread	4 years			X

A lot of this I can't remember for certain, but I am sure she was normal in everything except walking and talking.

SPEECH AND HEARING CLINIC

March 23, 1962

Parent's Name

Address

Dear——————:

We are sending you a report of our examination as you requested.

Your child's speech difficulty is characterized by an articulation problem and a word-finding "block." The factors responsible for these disorders are: (1) short auditory retention span, (2) visual-motor disturbance, (3) verbal aphasia, (4) ataxic tongue movements, (5) incipient stuttering. All, except the last factor, are probably a result of cerebral dysfunction. Another way to categorize her problem is: (1) cerebral palsy characterized by ataxic movements of the tongue, (2) perceptual deficiency characterized by the retention span and visual-motor disturbances, (3) expressive aphasia, and (4) incipient stuttering.

Short Auditory Retention Span

According to her chronological age, she should be able to repeat five or six numbers when they are presented to her in a sequence. She, at best, was able to repeat four numbers. Her performance with letters (when they were not arranged in an alphabetical sequence) was even poorer. Because of this impaired ability to retain that which she experiences through her auditory sense, she can be expected to have difficulty in language formulation which, after all, involves retaining the sound sequences that "make-up" words.

She can be helped by presenting four, five and six numbers and/or letter sequences to her and asking her to repeat them in the order presented (see enclosed pamphlet.) She is then expected to repeat this sequence in the proper order.

Example: *4 - 7 - 9 - 3, I repeat, 4 - 7 - 9 - 3*
3 - 5 - 1 - 9 - 2, I repeat, 3 - 5 - 1 - 9 - 2
1 - 7 - 2 - 2 - 8 - 1, I repeat, 1 - 7 - 2 - 2 - 8 - 1
A - C - F - C, I repeat, A - C - F - C and etc.

Note 1: *Be sure she can repeat the four number or four letter sequence before you start on the five sequence and etc.*

Note 2: *The reading examination that she took on February 23, 1962 indicated that her visual retention span (recall) was also impaired.*

Visual Motor

This impairment is characterized by her poor drawings which are not commensurate with her mental age. According to her father, she also has below-average ability when using her hands to "do things," such as batting a ball, etc.

Her inability to successfully cope with events that require seeing (visual) and doing (motor) might well be related to her reading problem; that is, there may be some disturbance in the feeding-back of information from the motor activities involved in reading to the visual sense required in reading.

Verbal Aphasia

Aphasia may be defined as an impairment in the ability to understand or use symbols. We think she understands what she hears, sees, or feels; she can also use graphic or written symbols fairly well. We do feel, however, that she is impaired in her ability to use verbal symbols. This impairment is characterized by what you explained as a "word-block." She knows what she wants to say, but can't seem to find the correct symbol to express herself.

Ataxic Tongue

We think that your daughter's articulation problem is caused by the incoordination of her speech musculature. This was evidenced by her poor response when we asked her to touch a tongue depressor (placed in different positions around her lips) with her tongue, and with her eyes closed.

Much help can be given to her by having her practice tongue exercises in front of a mirror; that is, touching various parts of her lips according to direction, or touching the handle of a spoon when placed in various positions around her lips. She should attempt to accomplish this task with her eyes closed; if she is unsuccessful, then she should try it again, looking in the mirror this time. Much laborious practice will be required but it will "pay off" in time.

Incipient Stuttering

Although there are no overt stuttering blocks, we do feel that your daughter is on the verge of becoming a stutterer. She manifested facial grimaces that were not too noticeable but still characteristic of mild stuttering. Usually such a response can be traced back to an environment loaded with pressures. Try to ease up on your demands, if possible.

We recommend a neurological examination, and then intensive speech therapy and remedial reading therapy this summer. We think we can also help educate you regarding the techniques and goals of the various types of therapy your child will need. You will then be able to help your daughter during the school year, when intensive therapy at our clinic is not feasible.

Sincerely,
Sol Adler, Ph.D., Director
Speech and Hearing Clinic

SA:jmp

READING CLINIC
ENGLISH DEPARTMENT
EAST TENNESSEE STATE COLLEGE

REPORT ON: Patient

                        Age   9 years   Grade   3
SCHOOL:
PARENTS: Name

                        Address
TEST ADMINISTERED: Durrell Analysis of Reading Difficulty
CLINICIAN:
TIME SPENT: Testing .... 1½ hours

                        Evaluation .... 4 hours

                        Conference with parents/teacher....½ hour

                        TOTAL HOURS..........................6 hours

Durrell Analysis of Reading Difficulty

A. Description of Tests

The *Analysis* consists of a series of tests and situations in which the examiner may observe in detail the various aspects of a child's reading. It covers a range in reading ability from the non-reader to the sixth-grade ability.

The primary purpose of the Analysis is to discover weaknesses and faulty habits in reading which may be corrected in a remedial program.

Each part of the *Analysis* has been standardized, thereby enabling the performance of one child to be considered and evaluated in light of typical performance of many children on a given grade level.

The following portions of the *Analysis* were administered:

1. Oral reading
2. Silent reading
3. Listening comprehension
4. Word recognition and word analysis
5. Letters
6. Sounds
7. Visual memory of words
8. Phonic spelling of words
9. Spelling test

B. Oral Reading

During this part of the test the child read while the examiner listened. In addition, a tape recording was made so that the oral reading could be evaluated more closely after the interview. The subsequent replays by the staff of the clinic aided in completing the diagnosis. After completing a selection on a grade level the child was asked to answer questions about what had been read. Responses to these questions provided the basis for measuring comprehension on each level.

The child read the first paragraph with seventy-five per cent comprehension and with a high first-grade rate. She made the following errors:

regressed on—Muff
                    is
                    a
                    little

called drinks—drink
        sleeps—sleep
        chair—hair

words pronounced for her—does
                            wet

On the second paragraph she read with eighty-three per cent comprehension and with a middle first-grade rate. The following errors were made by her:

regressed on—It
        to
        he

called began—getting
       black—blac
       went—wen
       wanted—want
       boy—boys
       did—could

omitted—a

words pronounced for her—tree
                    knew

On the third-grade selection, the child read with fifty-seven per cent comprehension and with a rate below the second grade. The following errors were made by her:

regressed on—Six
          boys
          their

called tent—ten
       side—si
       took—too
       things—time
       around—again
       went—was
       were—with
       bear—ba

omitted punctuation (one period)

words pronounced for her—river
                    afraid
                    thought

In summary, the child's comprehension was good through the second-grade level in oral reading while her rate of reading was a high first-grade level. Because of her many errors on easy words it is believed that her sight vocabulary is low and that her word-analysis ability is inadequate for third-grade work. She repeated words and phrases without any apparent pattern. Her phrasing was incorrect because she displayed extremely vocal and audible inhalation of air between words. She had difficulty answering questions dealing with "why," "how many," "where," and "what."

C. Silent Reading

During this part of the test the child read silently and was told to answer questions based upon what had been read. After reading a selection on a particular grade level, the child was asked to tell the examiner all that could be remembered about what had been read. (This comprehension check is referred to as *unaided recall* since the entire burden of remembering falls upon the child.) After the child has told all that could be remembered, questions were asked about any part of the selection omitted during unaided recall. Specific questioning about details serves to stimulate additional recall in many cases. (Since it is likely that a specific question will stimulate, this part of the comprehension measure is referred to as *aided recall.*)

The child's recall was so scanty that she was unable to be placed on any grade level in comprehension on the first, second, and third-grade paragraphs. Her rate of reading was above the second grade on the first and second paragraphs while her rate was the middle third-grade on the third paragraph. She displayed constant lip movements and whispering while reading silently. It was observed that she placed her book very close to her eyes while reading.

In summary, the child read with a middle third-grade rate of reading but was unable to comprehend what she read.

D. Listening Comprehension

During this part of the test the examiner read orally while the child listened. After a selection had been read the child was asked questions about what had been heard. The primary purpose of this part of the test was to learn whether the reading difficulty, if any, rested upon a lack of comprehension.

The child's listening comprehension was equal to a silent reading level of third grade. She had difficulty remembering the questions dealing with "what," "where," and "numbers."

E. Word Recognition and Analysis

This portion of the test is made up of two lists of words— one on the first grade reading level and the other on the second to sixth grades reading level. The word is flashed in front of the child and he is to tell you what he saw. Then if he misses, he may analyze the word for a few seconds and then tell you what he saw.

The child correctly identified on flash nineteen of the forty words in the first grade reading level list. This placed her on the high first-grade level. On analysis she identified correctly three additional words which gave her a grade placement of a middle first-grade level.

She could only identify correctly two of the fifty words on list two composed of words for grades two to six. This placed her on the low second-grade level. She made the following errors:

Word	She Called	Error
are	a	omitted the initial blend and final letter
children	church	omitted medial and final letters
around	come	substituted a more familiar word
love	live	substituted a medial letter
joy	just	substituted medial and final letters
bark	back	substituted a letter of a final blend
blow	blew	substituted a medial letter
please	pleasant	substituted a final ending
afraid	always	substituted medial and final letters
place	play	substituted final letter
ground	get	substituted a more familiar word
turkey	tur	omitted final ending
inch	inck	substituted final blend

She did not attempt the following words:

chair	other	cover	chimney	drink	strong
breakfast	lost	dark	road	different	stamp
fair	quickly	believe			

F. Letters—Naming, Matching, Identifying

The letters of the alphabet are arranged in a jumbled up order. The child must be able to name, match, and identify them both in capital form and in small letters.

The child omitted the letter "n" from the list of letters when asked to reproduce the alphabet. She was able to match and identify both capital and small letters in a jumbled order.

G. Visual Memory of Words—Primary

In this portion of the test you have twenty groups of words or letters. Each group contains similar words or letters. The child is flashed a word or letter and he must match it with one of the words or letters in the group. Since the only difference in some of the words within a group may be the one letter at beginning, medial, or ending of a suffix or prefix, the child must be alert and have good *visual perception.*

The child was able to reproduce eleven of the twenty words which placed her on a low first-grade level. Of her nine errors six were errors in the word ending and three errors in the medial letters. She had no difficulty with the beginnings of words.

H. Hearing Sounds in Words—Primary

This portion of the diagnosis is composed of twenty-nine groups of words, each group having something in common within itself. The child must have good auditory perception to accomplish this test successfully. Out of the three words in each group, he must select the one word that best sounds like the word the examiner repeated previously. He is forced to listen to initial and final sounds.

The child was able to reproduce twenty-eight of the twenty-nine words which placed her on the middle third-grade level. She failed to hear the ending "ic."

I. Sounds of Letters

During this test the child is to give the sounds of the phonograms or blends as they are shown to him.

The child did not know the sounds of the letters *m, l,*

ch, st, dr, tr, cl, pl, tw, sw, and *gr.* She had a tendency to place a vowel between the letters of the phonograms.

J. Phonic Spelling of Words

A list of fifteen words which are written exactly as they sound is given the child. The ability of the child to hear syllables, blends, vowels, and consonant sounds and reproduce them in writing is measured.

The child could not spell phonically any of the fifteen words which placed her below the fourth-grade level. She ommitted sounds and syllables, added sounds and syllables, used incorrect sounds, and reversed letters. She gave evidence of much insecurity.

K. Spelling Test

During this part of the test the child is asked to spell words common to his grade level in school.

The child was able to spell correctly four of the twenty words which placed her below the second-grade level. She omitted sounds and syllables, added sounds and syllables, used incorrect sounds, and reversed letters. She did not even attempt eight of the twenty words. She displayed marked insecurity in spelling.

L. Handwriting

The child's writing in the spelling part of the test and the writing of a paragraph is measured as to formation of the letters, slant, alignment, and crowding.

The child's handwriting displayed irregular heights and improper shapes and slants of letters.

SUMMARY OF READING ANALYSIS TESTS

M.

Test	Grade Placement	Grade Placement
1. Oral reading comprehension	second	Rate: high first
2. Silent reading comprehension	no level	Rate: middle third
3. Listening comprehension	third	
4. Word recognition	low second	
5. Word analysis	middle first	
6. Spelling	below second	
7. Sounds	middle third	
8. Phonic spelling of words	no level	
9. Visual memory of words	low first	

RECOMMENDATIONS

1. The child displays the ability to achieve on the third-grade level since she is able to comprehend on that level while listening. If she could read and understand what she reads, she could perform on the third-grade level, but she will need to develop a systematic method of word attack and to practice reading to achieve this level. At present she sacrifices understanding for speed in silent reading. In her oral reading she ignores her word errors and reads on, substitutes a more familiar word, guesses from the general forms, or waits for assistance. The following suggestions may be of help to her in developing her word recognition and analysis ability:

   a. Visual Analysis
      1. Look at the beginning, middle, and ending of the word to see if she recognizes any part.
      2. Look for little words in big words.
      3. Look for compound words.
      4. Learn simple initial sounds or prefixes, such as: *ab, ad, con, de, dis, ex, in, inter, mis, per, post, pre, pro, re, se, sub, trans,* and *un.*
      5. Learn simple endings such as: *al, ble, ad, er, es, est, ing, ous, ple,* and *tion.*

   b. Phonetic Analysis
      1. Learn the sounds of the long and short vowels.
      2. Learn the sound of the phonograms.
      3. Learn initial, medial and final blends.
      4. Listen for familiar sounds in words at the beginning, middle, and ending.
      5. Listen for the sounds on the endings of words and practice saying these sounds with the word.
      6. Learn and be able to apply the rules of syllabification. (Basic rules enclosed.)

2. The child needs to improve and expand the stock of words she can recognize on sight. Improvement will come with extensive silent reading for recreation, pleasure, and information on her part. She needs carefully planned additional exercises

and reading experiences designed to increase her sight vocabulary. As she reads silently, she must not speed through the material but concentrate on the words and the meanings of them. Someone should listen to her read easy material orally so as to call attention to her errors. She needs to learn and be able to recall the basic 220 words by Dolch.

3. For improvement of fluency, the child needs to recognize that words are written in thought units and should have practice in reading words in thought units. The workbook *Diagnostic Tests and Remedial Reading Exercises* by Leo J. Brueckner and William Dodge Lewis which is published by Holt, Rinehart, and Winston, Inc., 1010 Arch Street, Philadelphia 7, Pennsylvania, contains exercises which will be of help in developing fluency. The reading of easy, interesting material will aid in building the child's fluency. As the child reads orally she should be made conscious of the vocal inhalation which has become a habit with her and should try very hard to break this habit.

4. The child's spelling skills could be improved by following the steps listed below:

    a. Think about the whole word.
    b. Note any familiar letters or letter combinations at the beginning, in the middle, or at the end of the word.
    c. Say the word.
    d. Check the writing of the word.
    e. Write the word.
    f. Break into syllables that can be spelled easily.
    g. Make a column for each letter or letter combinations which give difficulty and fill the columns with words that contain the troublesome letters.
    h. Play word-building games—Anagrams, Junior Scrabble.

5. The child's slow reading rate, poor vocabulary, and lack of understanding of what is to be gained from the reading can be improved upon by consistent and conscientious practice. As a word by word reader, her comprehension will regularly increase when she learns how to improve her proficiency, to concentrate, and to concern herself with meaning rather than

with symbols on the page. She needs to be conscious of questions asking for who, when, where, or what of the material. She needs practice in recalling facts by sequence as they are listed in the reading material. Someone should ask her to retell the story she read to give her practice in recalling factual material in sequence. She should be encouraged to talk about what she has read. To break her habit of lip reading, a pencil may be placed between her teeth while she is reading silently.

6.   Reading is a combination of many skills. The child will need to learn each skill separately and to incorporate it into her reading. This transfer will not be difficult if she practices using each skill frequently. The most effective method is by establishing a special time (thirty to forty-five minutes) each day for reading easy, interesting, and informative materials both orally and silently. As her word recognition and analysis ability increases, the material she reads should increase in difficulty. Her confidence in her ability and her security should increase as her reading becomes more proficient. A visit to the library or to one of the bookshops should stimulate her interest in reading.

The following materials are recommended:

a. Phonics

1. *Phonics Skilltext,* Books A, B, and C, Charles E. Merrill Books, Inc., 1300 Alum Creek Drive, Columbus 16, Ohio.
2. Games—*What The Letters Say; Consonant Lotto; Vowel Lotto; Take; The Syllable Game;* and *Group Sounding Game,* The Garrard Press, Champaign, Illinois.

b. Basic Vocabulary and Diagnostic Reading

1. *Indian Folklore Series; Folklore of the World Series;* and *Pleasure Reading Books Series; Basic Vocabulary Series,* The Garrard Press, Champaign, Illinois.
2. *Enchanting Stories,* The John C. Winston Company, A division of Holt, Rinehart and Winston, Inc., 1010 Arch Street, Philadelphia 7, Pennsylvania.

c. Spelling

1. *My Word Book,* Book 2 and 3, Lyons and Carnahan, Atlanta, Georgia.

2. Workbook—*My Word Book,* Book 2 and 3, Lyons and Carnahan, Atlanta, Georgia.

3. *Helping Your Child With Spelling,* by Edward W. Dolch, Ph.D., The Garrard Press, Champaign, Illinois.

d. Pleasure Reading

1. *Foolish and Wise* followed by *Fun All Around,* Bobbs-Merrill Company, Inc., Indianapolis, Indiana.

2. *Fields and Fences* followed by *Town and Country,* Allyn and Bacon, Inc., New York, New York.

3. *Rachel Jackson, Tennessee Girl; Mary Mapes Dodge, Jolly Girl,* Bobbs-Merrill Company, Inc., Indianapolis, Indiana.

4. *The Boxcar Children; Mystery Ranch,* Scott, Foresman and Company, Atlanta, Georgia.

It was a pleasure to test this patient and if we can be of further assistance, please feel free to call upon us.

Yours very truly,

ALFG/lh

NEUROLOGICAL REPORT

April 19, 1962

Patient's Name

Address

CHIEF COMPLAINTS: Mild clumsiness and uncertainty and unsteadiness of gait.
Mild speech handicap.

PRESENT ILLNESS: This nine year old white female patient has exhibited a history of very mildly retarded progress, both physically and intellectually since birth. A review of her past history indicates that she weighed some seven pounds three ounces at birth, following a full-term, normal pregnancy except for intermittent vaginal bleeding, but no other unusual abnormalities. She was delivered by breech presentation and apparently some problem arose with respect to prolapse of the cord during delivery, and she was quite cyanotic at the time of birth and was placed in an incubator with oxygen for a period of about three days. She remained in the hospital for a period of about ten days, but with improvement was returned home.

Subsequently, her development was a bit slow with the child first beginning to hold her head at two months of age, sitting alone at eight months, standing at twelve months of age, and walking at seventeen months of age, and talking at twenty-four months of age. At the age of about three years, as a result of persistent slight difficulty in walking, bilateral tendon achilles tenotomies and bilateral Grice's procedures for pes planus were carried out by Dr. . . . . , ... , ... , Subsequently, the child has always appeared a bit clumsy on her feet and has walked in somewhat an awkward fashion, and falls frequently and is unable to run quite as fast as other children. She has proven to be left handed and the family seems to attribute this largely to the fact that she has always been able to use her left hand and arm a bit better perhaps than the right. There is no family history of left handedness. For a period of three months, she experienced seizures and has had measles, chicken pox, mumps, and in December 1961, a tonsillectomy. She is at the present time encountering a great deal of difficulty with reading in school, but apparently does fairly well with most of her other school work.

At the present time, the mother reports that she seems to encounter difficulty in expressing herself with speech, particularly in finding a proper choice of words. She does not write as well as the mother feels she should, but seems to believe this is attributable to some clumsiness of her hands and fingers and she does not color too well, but is fairly adequate. She has previously been examined at the Speech and Hearing Clinic of Tennessee State College in Johnson City, Tennessee where it was felt that she had both impairment of visual-motor coordination, and expressive dysphasia and dysarthria largely secondary to ataxia or poor control and coordination of tongue and palatal musculature. Speech therapy and remedial reading have been advised.

EXAMINATION: The general physical and neurological examination disclose the presence of an affable, alert, quite well developed white female patient who appears in quite good contact. Her attention span is short and her attention is difficult to attain and to maintain. She is a bit flighty and distractible and seems to encounter mild difficulty in concentrating. She exhibits a very obvious restriction in quick successive movements of the tongue, and poor control and coordination of the tongue and palatal musculature. She exhibits dysarthria and apparently a very evident expressive mild dysphasia in the sense that at times even in naming objects, she encounters difficulty in finding a proper word to accurately name an object yet seems to understand quite well its intent and purpose in usefulness. There is present moderate spasticity involving both upper and lower extremities, and apparently maximal in the lower extremities, with generalized hyper-reflexia and bilateral extensor-plantar responses. Her gait is a bit awkward and mildly wide-based, with the patient walking partially with knee flexion bilaterally, running clumsily and awkwardly in a similar fashion to her walking. There is reduction in quick successive movements of both arms and legs. There is moderate dyspraxia in both hands, noted particularly with safety pin test and perhaps slightly more marked on the right than on the left side. There is no obvious demonstrable sensory deficit.

IMPRESSION: Cerebral spastic disease, manifested by spastic tetraparesis, probably maximal in her lower extremities. She exhibited as well dysarthria and in addition an expressive type dysphasia of mild degree, undoubtedly related to damage to speech centers in the left hemisphere. Her cerebral palsy is very likely related to inadequate oxygenation either during delivery or probably more likely during the prolonged period of recurrent vaginal bleeding during gestation.

RECOMMENDATIONS: This child probably could benefit considerably by prolonged periods of speech therapy, particularly with some adequate instruction in procedures and techniques that might be followed up at home by the parents. She was advised to return to Johnson City for further follow-up care, and if arrangements could not be made there, that arrangements could be made here at the Rehabilitation Hospital for out-patient speech therapy and instruction during the summer months.

ATC:nwj

cc: Dr.

Dr.

Dr. Sol Adler

FINAL CASE SUMMARY

PATIENT'S NAME   SPEECH & HEARING THERAPIST:

ADDRESS: (STUDENT REPORT)

SPEECH THERAPY
DYSARTHRIA

Due to dysarthria, characterized by sluggish tongue movements, tongue exercises were initiated. The patient also received some articulation therapy, particulary on the blends, but this has not been very successful and will not be until tongue movements are more proficient. I introduced the tongue exercises then turned them over to the mother to perform at home.

SHORT RETENTION SPAN

I began working with the patient to increase her retention span by reading very simple stories and questioning her about the contents following each paragraph. We advanced to the point where she could respond successfully to questions asked at the completion of an entire story. She is now ready for more complex stories.

She had a difficult time retaining more than three numbers when they were in random order. She could, however, do much better when the numbers were in ascending order—and has been able to successfully recall five numbers in this manner.

EXPRESSIVE APHASIA

The patient's most urgent problem is that of her word finding difficulty. I have experimentally tried several procedures with her in order to discover the most desired method. She forgets names of everyday objects, and in conversation cannot express herself.

I find that the method of building up association and relationship through means of her concept formulation is most successful in approaching this aphasic problem.

The following techiniques have been used:

1. Began naming objects, i.e., animals, utensils, clothes, etc. and discussed the function of each. Even if she knew the name of the object, we discussed it thoroughly anyway. This procedure was for the purpose of showing her how to think of all the relationships with each object so that its name would be easier to derive.

2. Proceeded to work with pictures that had a common relationship. She was not pressured for the name at this time. The important factor was for her to think of the association. For example, the relationship of a blanket to a bed.

3. Next, worked for the names of these pictures by using the method described in step 1. It was much easier for her to arrive at the name after she had discussed the function and relationship of the pictures with me.

4. Picked pictures at random and she had to group them according to their relationship. (For example, apple, orange, potato, chair, bed, carrots, dog, and horse.) This exercise was successful only after she had thought of the association of the objects.

5. Without visual clues, I then read to her a list of objects and she had to tell me the association between them, i.e., bicycle and car, toothbrush and teeth.

6. Worked on naming pictures, per se. I used pictures of everything I could find—clothes, food, animals, furniture, etc. Whenever she had any difficulty naming we would go all through the association method again and also with

the relationships on the board. Usually she had little trouble in finding the name after the above procedure. When she did get the correct name, I let her make up a sentence using the word, then she wrote it. This was to help reinforce the word or name.

7. Began to work on picture-name relationships. Clues were given only when necessary at which time only the initial sound was given. Much progress was noted in this area.

8. Worked on sequence formation. This was again the process of association. I would tell a story to her and then she had to put the sequence puzzle together by means of sequential thinking. Then she would have to tell me the story. This procedure was also good for retention.

REMARKS:

As is indicated, I began helping her verbally through the association process and gave her the name of the object or picture. Then I advanced her to the stage of thinking mentally with some speed in order to produce the correct name. This was proving very successful and she was beginning to name every thing with little difficulty.

I began working in simple and concrete stages and gradually began to move toward more advanced and abstract levels of performance.

BEHAVIOR:

The patient was a delightful child to work with. She was always cheerful and cooperative. I gained excellent rapport with her and our clinician-patient-parent relationship was very good. The mother was most cooperative and my instructions were always carried out to the best of her ability. I instructed the mother in how to work with the child and I am sure that due to intense interest, understanding and motivation, she will do her utmost to help her daughter.

FINAL CASE SUMMARY

PATIENT'S NAME   SPECIAL EDUCATOR:

ADDRESS

PERCEPTUAL TRAINING

Perceptual training with the child has been concentrated in these areas: figure ground-relationships, visual-motor activities, and finer visual discrimination, all of which, however, overlap in varying degrees. Difficulties are not gross but they are involved in many learning situations.

Part of the child's difficulty is due to the fact that she "jumps to conclusions." She takes a quick look at the design she is to compare or copy, sees the major outlines, and guesses at the rest. When she voluntarily looks again, she is often able to correct her own error. When she *doesn't* take a second look, if she is told that there is something not quite right about her work, she can almost invariably correct her own mistake, discovering it independently.

Her habit of constantly erasing her written work has decreased considerably since she has begun to observe more carefully and more accurately *before* attempting to write.

Quite a bit of chalkboard work has been done, using at first templates for the circle and square figures, and progressing to free-hand drawing of these in numerous combinations with lines. Dot-to-dot work here was concentrated largely on learning to cross and recross lines she had previously drawn. At first she completely avoided crossing the line, going completely around it; later she was able to cross, but with a bent line; she is now able to draw a reasonably straight line under these conditions, although once recently she reverted to complete avoidance, saying, "I can't cross the line." However, she can ordinarily perform so well in this task that she is able to draw a star without once removing her chalk from the board, thus:

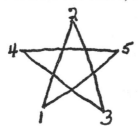

An attack was made on the figure-ground difficulty through the use, at first, of large colored silhouettes on a white background, gradually increasing the background strength through shades of buff and then gray, and finally to figured and then to graph paper. Meanwhile, the foreground image was changed to black and gradually decreased in size and increased in complexity, until she could handle with ease designs made with a felt-tip pen or ball point pen or even pencil. She remarked, though, that designs on gray or buff backgrounds are easier to see than those on graph paper because the latter is "white."(!)

Practice in visual-motor skills was given through coloring and cutting of simple designs, making pipe cleaner objects, folding paper on which a design was first traced and then cut to make a border pattern, folding a napkin to make a flower cup-holder. These were activities that she enjoyed very much, but she needs additional practice of this type to increase her level of performance.

Finer visual discrimination was a prime goal this summer, and since it is impossible to separate this from figure-ground and visual-motor activities, a great deal of time was spent in this area.

The child was asked to copy letter combinations involving such series as TVAI, MWVA, etc. in a mixture of sizes; to select from many examples the letters *b* and *d*, which she frequently reverses; to copy letter combinations involving these letters and all the vowels; to select samples of SAW and WAS, which she often also reverses . . . all of these in an attempt to encourage closer inspection of the order in which these letters occur.

Fine discrimination was required in matching a number of different kinds of real sea shells with colored pictures in books with the small ones on her bracelet. In this activity she performed very well.

Since she frequently misses the middle or end of the words she reads, considerable work was done on comparing strips of designs (again on an increasingly stronger background and weaker foreground) to find the duplicate of each. All were similar except for a small detail near the middle or end of the strip, although the position of the different one varied, sometimes coming first. It was, therefore, necessary for her to scrutinize every *part,* as well as the whole.

Although there appears to be considerable improvement in each of the areas in which we worked, a continuation of this type of activity would be profitable, I feel, increasing its difficulty as she obtains mastery. Therefore, I am suggesting to her mother the following types of activities for further practice.

1. Games involving matching cards, such as Animal Rummy, Crazy 8's or better still, homemade ones similar to the ones we used in individual work.

2. Commercial games like checkers or Chinese checkers, to help her distinguish the foreground from a strong background.

3. Activities in which she will have to distinguish between:

$$m \ldots \ldots \ldots \ldots \ldots n$$
$$0 \ldots \ldots \ldots u \ldots \ldots v$$
$$b \ldots \ldots \ldots \ldots \ldots d \text{ (perhaps adding p)}$$

4. Matching a figure or row of figures with its exact duplicate, but either larger or smaller.

5. Use of strips of letters or designs, including one or more variants:

h h h h h h h h h h d h h h h d h h h
h b h h h b h h b (etc.)
m m m m n m m m m n m n m m
x x x z x x z x x x z x x z

6. Tracing designs, using tracing paper.

7. Tracing designs, using a cardboard pattern.

8. Coloring pictures.

9. Cutting pictures.

10. Reproducing designs of increasing complexity.

With continued practice in these areas, I am quite sure that the child can make a considerable amount of further progress.

It was a pleasure to work with the child and her mother. They are remarkable people.

FINAL CASE SUMMARY

PARENTS' NAME   REMEDIAL READING THERAPIST:

ADDRESS

REMEDIAL READING

Dear . . . . :

Your child has been enrolled in our Reading Clinic for the Summer. This is the final report on her work. The following paragraphs were written by the Clinician who worked with your child. A copy of this report, the daily logs, as well as the initial diagnosis will be on file in the offices of the Clinic. It is our hope that this report will give you an insight into the work and its results with your child.

A study of the results of the diagnostic reading test revealed that she needed help with the following: 1. oral and silent reading comprehension; 2. silent reading; 3. listening comprehension; 4. word recognition; 5. spelling; 6. sounds. The following evaluation gives a description of what was done in each area, the progress made and suggestions for future work.

Listening Comprehension: Your child's span of attention needs to increase in length of time. I began by reading very short selections and asking questions of the who, what type. This proved to be most rewarding because it wasn't too long before she could retell a story in proper sequence. Sequence gave her trouble at first. She would jump from beginning to end and back again. By the end of the session she could even rearrange jumbled sentences in the correct order. I increased the difficulty of material read and she could recall the correct answer or retell the story.

Suggestions: It would be helpful if some one would read daily to her for a short time. Different types of material should be selected and it should be both fact and fiction. She should be allowed to choose some of these stories. The stories need to be broken into parts unless they are short ones. Always remember to check by means of thought questions. There are other ways of checking also. Ask her to give a list of characters, give words to describe the one she likes best, true-false statements, or sentences where she completes the meaning with a key word. Perhaps she may progress to the point where she could draw a picture to illustrate something she remembered. She needs to do this activity perhaps not everyday but at least twice a week.

Oral Reading: She cannot be expected to read fluently because of the difficulty she has with her articulation. I noticed a great improvement in speech and the improvement in her speech and the improvement in her reading were very noticeable.

I used a great deal of material from the books she was reading for pleasure. The conversational parts were most helpful. Often we took different parts or I would be the book and she would read the conversation.

The same type of questions used for listening comprehension were used for oral reading. She has a good memory and her recall of facts is also good. She never wants you to tell her the answer to a question. She would say, "don't tell me, please let me try." If you reread the paragraph and told her to listen for the answer she could always find it.

One cause of her low rate in reading was because she did not know her two hundred and twenty basic words. She knows them now and this has brought about a marked increase in rate.

Suggestions: When the child took a final test on her basic words, as I have said, she knew all but about twelve. If this is to be a permanent learning she will need to continue some form of drill work. The flash card technique will not work with her and it is a waste of time to use it. I used two boxes of Dolch's Basic Sight Vocabulary Cards (The Garrard Press, Champaign, Illinois) arranged in alphabetical order. She matched the cards saying the words as she made her books of two cards. Another way is to take all the cards of one letter, spread them out and then match using the second pile for this. This is of no value unless the word is pronounced as it is matched.

Silent Reading Comprehension: She is reading in thought units. She had formed the habit of word-by-word reading. We practiced on seeing more than one word. Material blocked off in thought units was very helpful. In this type of material a line separates the thought units and you read from line to line. Her comprehension was always good. If she knows she will be answering questions after she reads she tries harder. Sometimes she does not read all the material when she reads silently. There too it is better if she reads short selections with questions following each reading. Retelling its story is also good for check on comprehension.

Suggestions: She needs to continue to read for pleasure, books for the most part of her own choosing. This will help her build up her stock of sight words and give her practice of the basic vocabulary. She loves to read library books and some of this needs to be done silently. Library books also serve the purpose of providing material for oral reports. This she does quite well. One way of building up the stock of sight words is to use a definite word attack technique. If she would follow the steps in the following outline it would be helpful in unlocking words:

1. Look at word carefully.
2. Do you see any known part?
3. Look at the beginning, the middle, the ending.
4. How many parts do you hear?
5. Do you see any little words in it?
6. How many vowels?
7. Try to divide the word into syllables.
8. Do you see a suffix, a prefix?
9. See if you can pronounce the word.
10. If you can't pronounce it look it up in the dictionary.
11. Last of all ask for help.

Spelling: She displays marked insecurity in spelling according to results of a spelling test given in the Clinic. To be proficient in spelling one must be able to hear syllables, blends, vowels and consonant sounds and reproduce them in writing. This is hard for her to do. She was adept at dividing words into syllables and she is able to follow some of the basic rules for syllabication. She needed to use a plan for spelling not dependent on sound.

I used the one described below. It was a combination of many but it worked.

Suggestions: I usually selected her spelling words from ones in her reading that she did not know. The steps followed were as follows:

1. Look at the whole word carefully.
2. How does it begin?
3. How does it end?
4. Notice the middle part.
5. Say the word slowly.
6. Write the word using link-letter (separate letters on small cards that fit together).
7. Write the word on the chalk-board (or on large sheets of paper). Pronounce the word as you write.
8. With your finger trace the word and pronounce it as you do so.
9. Repeat No. 8.
10. Close your eyes. Do you see it with your mind's eye?
11. Write word on paper, pronounce as you write.
12. Check your word.
13. If it is correct write the word in a sentence.

This is a little tedious but it worked with her. The first word she learned to spell was "telephone" and every day she insisted on writing it again. After a short time, possibly, you would not need all these steps. Before too long the visual-auditory steps would be all that was needed. That would be—see the word—hear the word—write it from memory.

Comments:

She requires individual help. For a time she will possibly not do too well in a group. She needs to read books on her own level of performance. She has made exceptional progress this summer session. If she can continue to have individual help it is not going to be too long before she will be able to do successful work in her class. Long assignments frustrate her. Too many spelling words confuse her. Right now ten words per week would be enough.

She lacks self-confidence. This needs to be built up. She needs to do things in class that she can do well and thus bring recognition of her true worth. It would help to give reports on books she has read, report on trips she has taken. She can't take pressure, neither can she hurry with her work. Praise she needs and deserves. It works like a charm. She works best in an atmosphere of friendly understanding.

The experience of working with this child was a delightful one. She was ambitious, cooperative, cheerful and happy. We became good friends and I will always remember our happy summer.

Should you desire a conference with us, we shall be glad to arrange for it.

Very sincerely yours,

INDEX